Heal You.....

*The Remarkable Journeys of
Ordinary People
Healing Themselves of Dis-ease
in Extra Ordinary Ways*

MEDICAL DISCLAIMER

The information provided in this book does not substitute for professional medical advice.

Please consult a medical professional or healthcare provider if you need medical advice, diagnoses, or treatment.

The author and contributors are not liable for risks or issues associated with using or acting upon the information in this book.

Dedication

I dedicate this book to anyone and everyone suffering dis-ease.

May this book help you find a way to heal yourself.

Introduction

This book not only shows that what we are told with regards to self-healing being impossible may be wrong but explores and showcases examples of real people proving this.

Taking responsibility for our own health is more important than ever in today's society where physically visiting a doctor is becoming increasingly difficult, hospitals are cancelling more and more elective surgeries and the cost of conventional treatments is ever escalating, not only in financial terms but also the long-term health cost of taking pharmaceuticals.

Heal Yourself details a wide variety of people from different backgrounds, who have decided to step outside the box of so-called conventional medicine and treatments, to take back responsibility for themselves and their health, by embarking on self-healing journeys. They achieve this by using various non-pharmaceutical interventions and techniques that are more in harmony with a natural state of well-being.

This book dedicates a complete chapter to each person, exploring their individual journey along with their personal stories, in their own words, of how their dis-ease impacted their life and how they took control of their situation to bring themselves back to wellness, with the intention of inspiring others to do the same.

These people were told by their doctors that their conditions are "chronic, life-long and life-threatening", yet, they have miraculously self-healed or are healing.

I hope our stories help you to start your healing journey back to wellness.

Acknowledgements

I would not have been able to write this book without the support of my wonderful husband. He has supported me physically, emotionally, mentally, spiritually and financially, not only throughout my dark days and healing but in my every day. Whilst we had a difference of opinion on healing at times, he gave me the space I needed, to do what I needed.

I want to thank my family too, for their support over the years. I know that my suffering was tough on them.

And last but by no means the least, I want to say a HUGE thank you to all the healers who have freely donated their healing to this book, with the sole purpose of helping other people to heal too. May you all be blessed with good health for the rest of your lives.

Contents

7

Part One – My Journey

"When we experience for ourselves, or witness in another person, something that we've once believed to be impossible, we are freed in our beliefs to transcend those limitations in our own lives"

Dr Joe Dispenza.

Foreword

I t is oftentimes out of our greatest despair, that we can turn inward and find solutions to seemingly impossible situations. It is an inescapable fact that we have a choice to create health or dis-ease of the mind, body, and spirit. Because of one of the most recognized laws of the universe, the law of cause and effect, every decision we make has a reward or consequence. Everything we think, say, and do has a direct effect on our life!

In our world today, misinformation is abundant. People all over the world are sick and dying from doing nothing wrong. They are misled by propaganda and advertising. The medical industry is ready and willing to prescribe medication, surgeries, and toxic therapies for anything that may ail a person. The truth is, we are created as a self-healing being. Our body is capable of miraculous healing on an epic level!

In my own personal experience, I have witnessed first-hand how convincing medical advice can be. I have healed myself from emotional trauma, after the loss of nearly every family member. Despite my doctor's advice to use prescription medication to fight the symptoms of depression, I found that prayer and meditation healed my challenges, rather than merely remedying the symptoms. My story, along with many others, are what makes this book so unique.

In Sarah Dawkins' beautifully written book, you will read many incredible stories of ordinary people who have naturally healed their body of multiple health issues of the mind, body, and spirit. Sarah shares how she overcame her own health challenges, thus inspiring her book.

As you read through each story, you will discover that many were given a grim diagnosis. All these people recognized a need for healing, and began their wellness journey. Despite what doctors had told them, each remarkable story shares how they took matters into their own hands.

This book gives you, the reader, a clear blueprint of how each person over-came their specific health challenges. Many healed without the use of medication or doctor intervention, while other healers reduced their medications throughout their healing journeys, some to be free of medication and others to be almost free of it. My hope is that you will feel inspired and empowered to embark on your own self-healing journey!

To your health and vitality.

Diana Martin-Gotcher, Ph.D.

Published Author & Speaker

www.Thrive-DianaPhD.com

The Power to Heal

A powerful subject in itself, tackled head on by Sarah Dawkins, who believes in the power of the mind, alternative medicines and your own supremacy to believe. Sarah a very talented lady who practices what she teaches.

Why I ask, shouldn't the human body be able to heal itself? If one loses a finger nail another one grows – and why? Because you believe it will. If you scratch or bruise yourself the body will restore to normal.

In the sporting world athletes taking part train hard to reach the pinnacle of their performance, it is the same with footballers and other sports, teaching their muscles to respond at the highest level. The pain that goes with it - they know will go away.

The body is a fortress with an immune system to protect it. My belief is it needs training similar to other activities. The difference is, it is a mental exercise to destroy thoughts or learnings that have been mis-taught.

From early in life, we are told we will become infirm and have difficulty getting about. The brain believes it. But is it true?

I am nearing ninety and write regularly for a newspaper and my darling wife is not far behind me. Twelve years ago, she was diagnosed with arthritis in her knees, the doctor told her there was nothing he could do, just keep taking the pain killers. Today she walks without pain, or pain killers and with the sheer belief it is possible to heal.

My mother in-law was in her late seventies and after an illness, she was struggling to get about and was using walking sticks. She wanted a wheelchair. It was hard but we said "No." She discarded the walking sticks and for the rest of her life, walked upright until she died at ninety.

We wish Sarah Dawkins well in her teachings of a difficult subject. In this well written book, she confirms her own thoughts by listening to others' experiences, that it is possible with the right attitude to one's own ability, to live in harmony with yourself.

Percy Chattey

Author and writer

Preface

Many years ago, I was told by a "gifted" friend that I would write a book. I didn't really believe her because, at the time, as I was in a dark abyss and suffering from depression. I had nothing to write about...and besides which, I was just a nobody! Still, I held onto the notion as I trusted and respected her.

About a year after this conversation, I was well on the way out of the suicidal depression I had been in for a few years and this book started around ten years ago, solely as my journey of self-healing naturally. My reason for writing it was to help other people understand that there is light at the end of the tunnel and it is possible to heal without pharmaceuticals.

As I got further into my book, I felt something was missing, it was just about me, my life, the depression I suffered and how I healed myself. How was this going to help many people? It seemed very egocentric. I questioned my purpose for writing it. Was it because I wanted to be a writer? Was it because I wanted to boost my ego? Honestly, at that time, while I wanted to help others, I was also a people pleaser, (a known trauma response). I wasn't really sure of my "why", other than to "help people", so I walked away from it, leaving it to sit on my computer whilst I figured it out.

Five years later, I had a bit of a revelation... At last, I understood! Many people are suffering unnecessarily in the world because they are stuck in the medical model system, reliant on doctors and pharmaceutical drugs to help improve their symptoms and ameliorate the dis-ease (I'd seen plenty as a Nurse!) I realised that many of these people didn't know that they needed to heal the root cause of the symptoms, or how to start their own healing. I felt that they needed information to take back the responsibility for their health...and with a plan, they could kick start themselves into healing the health conditions and dis-eases they were struggling with.

I could help *more* people by documenting *many* people's healing journeys, from *many* health conditions, not just my own. Of course, at first, I was unsure how to do this or what it would look like, so I spent an inevitable couple of years floundering, not knowing how to move this book forward...unsure of the best way to get this important message out there. So, I decided to concentrate my efforts on my business, until I had a better idea of how to do it. I grew my business and did well, earning awards as a local and national entrepreneur, within the UK. However, deep inside, the itch remained...this book needed to be written!

Then out of the blue, I woke up one day with the thought that I just have to make this work and needed to think bigger... much bigger! I started putting requests out, initially through Facebook, asking for healers and miraculously, I received a couple of responses. These beautiful souls shared their healing with me. I was in awe of their outer and inner work and their journeys were truly inspiring.

Then self-doubt crept in and I wondered if it was just pie in the sky and if my book would ever come to fruition. Who the hell did I think I was? Writing a book? Publishing a book? What was I thinking? I must have been crazy to think I could. There was no way this was going to happen, so again, I just put it to bed on my computer.

As I did more inner work and healing, I started to understand my negative mind chatter and the need to heal my mental, emotional and spiritual bodies as well as my physical body. Doing this helped boost my confidence and (almost) silence the "negative-nelly" on my shoulders, whispering in my ears. I got to a point where I realised and understood why and what was going on. I changed my thoughts (because I am not my thoughts) and began again... But this time with gusto!

I signed up to more social media platforms, joined health-related groups and put out more requests. I HAD to get this book written!

Many healers came forwards wanting to share their healing. Every one of them unique and ALL as important as each other. To try and keep it so that no one healer stood out more than any other, I requested everyone to average their word count to around one thousand words. I also asked the healers in this book to write about their diagnosis or diagnoses, symptoms and specifically how they healed, so that the readers could not only relate but also so they could try the same things, to heal themselves.

I then told them that I couldn't pay for their healing journeys, they would have to be donated. Just about all of the people I spoke to were happy to give the information without anything back in return, solely to help others. Many of these people who healed are coaches because they too wanted to help others after they healed themselves. I found a small way that I could help them and it was for the healers to add their contact details if they chose to. This way, if any reader wanted more information, they would be able to get in touch with the healer that they resonated with.

To try and get a variety of healers, I then started undertaking targeted searches of dis-eases that I had only one or no healers for. There were people out there and I started reaching out to them individually. When I told these people the reason for my book, they wanted to come on board. It was just exhilarating. So many people wanting to help others to start their own healing, without asking for anything in return. I was totally overwhelmed by the generosity of so many people.

As people sent me their healing journeys, I realised there was a need to edit some, for grammar, flow and to remove colloquialisms, to make sure readers from anywhere in the world would understand what was being said. However, I have left spellings in American-English because they are correct for the writer.

So here is *Heal Yourself,* a book of healers, healing dis-eases that many were told were incurable, life-long and life-threatening, proving beyond a doubt that we CAN heal ourselves and highlighting the many ways.

Lastly, I'd just like to thank everyone I have spoken to and who has responded to my requests. The response has been overwhelming and I am still getting people approaching me to share their journey. I had to have a cut-off point to get this book published and out into the world to start helping people, so for that reason, it is highly likely that there will be a second volume in the not-too-distant future, highlighting the incredible self-healing journeys of even more wonderful and amazing people!

At the back of this book, I have listed each contributor's name and contact information where they have given their permission so that you the reader, can contact them directly about their individual journey, should you wish to.

I have also included a – rather long – glossary of terms, to help you to understand the medical terms and healing treatments used by some of the healers.

Finally, if you want to contact me to discuss this book, its contents or simply have a chat about healing then you can email me at **SarahDawkins@pm.me**

Alternatively, my website is at **www.SarahDawkins.com.** Here you will find further information about me and what I do.

Please enjoy this book and while you are reading it consider the personal bravery each person summoned up from within themselves to step out of the box and take the first steps on their incredible journeys...a step every person can take, if they so choose to do so.

Who Am I

I am Sarah Dawkins. Coach, Nurse, Wife, Mother...and Self-Healer.

You could describe my childhood as a rollercoaster of events and emotions. Both my parents were skilled; my mother a nurse and my father a fireman and I truly believe they both wanted the best for both myself and my younger sister.

I was born in 1964, in a small deprived town in Northern Britain and, before I was of school age, my parents were separated and divorced. I spent some time after their divorce living with my uncle's family, my sister and my father. Eight of us in a tiny, two up, two down, mid-terraced house, with myself, sister, father and two male cousins, all sleeping in the attic. I had little or no privacy.

Although we lived apart from our mother, she would come for visits and take us out for some time. Shunting between parents, the visits were highly emotionally charged and at times, ended in tears. My mother remarried and I got on well with my new stepfather.

It was when I was around the age of seven, my father remarried. He, along with my new stepmother, my sister and myself moved into a new family home. While I had slightly more personal space as I now only shared a bedroom with my sister and not four other people.

Sometime in the summer months, when I was about nine years old, I was sexually abused by an elderly male neighbour. I was a very naïve child, so I didn't understand what was happening or why.

Whilst I had a good brain, I didn't like school and as a result, my report always said: "Sarah could do better". I attended three different high schools through circumstance, but it was at the first one, Grammar School, where I was regularly bullied by three girls. My life felt pretty tough then and I was reduced to tears through fear almost every day.

At the age of fourteen, I left my father and stepmother's house, to live with my mother and stepfather, moving to another "new life".

I now had my very own bedroom (personal space at last) and a comparative abundance of material things but emotionally this period was just as difficult. Now I was a teenage girl in the full throes of puberty and carrying all the extra baggage that entailed. However, I suppose you could say I had now found a fairly "normal" middle-class life.

Leaving school at sixteen to work was liberating and suddenly I could do more of what I wanted. Still, I was living at home and had to abide by the house rules, which I found difficult and restrictive.

On my seventeenth birthday, I left home to live on my own, working long hours, playing and drinking hard and smoking. I was rebelling on a grand scale. I was fiercely independent and did what I wanted and when I wanted.

Suddenly, out of the blue, my stepfather died after a short fight with bowel cancer, when I was eighteen. He was only forty-four and had been healthy and full of life. It hit me hard, I was devastated. Following his death, I became bulimic, binge eating out of control, then vomiting, trying to control my emotions and weight. My weight ballooned. This was another problem I dealt with on my own.

At nineteen, there were more promises of living "a good life", this time by a prospective employer, which led to a move to the south coast of England. This promise left me pregnant and unmarried at twenty-one. The father of my unborn child and his family wanted me to have an abortion because of their orthodox background. I could not go through with the trauma of ending a life and this left our relationships strained.

Whilst pregnant with my son, my cousin (who we had lived with) died suddenly of a burst ulcer, aged twenty-one. I recall travelling back to the north of England for the funeral with a heavy heart and a heavy belly. Any funeral is emotional, but with super-charged emotions from my pregnancy, I found it incredibly difficult.

As a young single parent, hundreds of miles from my family and any chance of support, I struggled with my mental health, induced by my circumstances. Eventually, I moved back up to the northwest of England, to be nearer to my family. My mother married again and I got on well with my new stepfather.

My life at this stage, although difficult as a single parent with no financial support from my son's father, seemed to settle down somewhat and I met my now-husband. After an initially difficult start to married life and my husband's return to full time, higher education without financial support, I had to work several jobs to try and support us.

During this period, I experienced a sexual assault at the hands of someone I trusted. I kept this to myself for decades, to protect the people I loved.

Halfway through my husband's time at university, I was pregnant again. During this pregnancy my grandmother died suddenly from a stroke. I found myself again grieving for another relative whilst there was a new life growing inside me. Never again was I going to get pregnant!

Our daughter was born; another mouth to feed with even less money. However, once my husband finished his degree, he got a good job offer on the other side of the country. Another move to another new life. This time was different, I now had a stable family life, we had a bit of money and a nice home. Maybe now I could find and be myself.

I started my Nurse training in 1998 and loved it. I worked hard and attained good marks. Then, during my second year, my mother-in-law died of cancer and my second stepfather died of a sudden stroke. At this time, my relationship with my mother was very strained so I didn't attend his funeral. I deeply regret this decision.

In 2001, I qualified as a Registered Nurse. Yet, I didn't feel that I was good enough. I still felt I had to "prove" myself worthy, to myself and my family. This led to me undertaking a post-graduate degree of BSc (Hons) in nursing but it didn't give me the satisfaction I thought it would.

We moved to the USA in 2004, obtaining family green cards after I passed the exam to work as a nurse there. We sold everything for the experience of living and working in a different country (having been there several times on holiday). Sadly, it wasn't anything like I believed it would be, so, two years later, we returned to the UK, buying a house from the internet without even seeing it.

The feeling of not being good enough pushed me into undertaking a master's degree (MSc). During my MSc, I went through some very troubling times that, even after my childhood traumas, led to my darkest days. I spiralled into a deep and dark, depression, began to drink in excess and became suicidal. I refused the antidepressants prescribed by my doctor as I believed there had to be another way to heal.

I was referred to a counsellor, who was concerned about my lack of self-care. My family were also seriously concerned but I didn't see it. I saw nothing but the darkness of the abyss I was in.

Anyway, here I am, some years later, alive and with a good life at last. My husband and I have a lovely home, the kids are now grown up, left home and are self-supportive. Now that I have healed, I am at peace with myself and the world. I am no longer filled with black thoughts of suicide nor view the world as a battleground.

Whilst I understand that everyone has problems of some kind in their lives, it seemed as though I had more than my fair share of issues and health problems. That said, I don't doubt that there are people who have been through and still going through problems larger than mine.

This book details how I finally realised that we can heal ourselves if we truly want to and I share mine and others' natural, self-healing journeys.

I hope all our healing inspires you to embark on your own healing journey, culminating in the enjoyment of improved and vibrant health.

Love, light and blessings to you all.

My Life Through Adversity to Healing and Success

Throughout my childhood years,
There were shed many tears.
A broken home at age three,
living with dad, sister and uncle D

Given a new family at seven,
I found it a difficult lesson.
Experienced sexual abuse at nine.
This was a need in others, not mine.

Harsh bullying followed at eleven,
feeling very low with a lack of expression.
A different family and city at fourteen,
and a real promise of living the dream.

Out of this home at seventeen,
all unreal, feeling an in-between.
An encounter and pregnant at twenty-one,
gazing in wonder at the new life just begun.

Heart's desire and wedded bliss at twenty-six.
Feeling happy and becoming quite the eccentric.
Sexual assault at twenty-eight,
Many years of hiding it, full of hate.

Some joy in motherhood again at thirty.
Studying, two degrees, but feeling rather dirty.
A bottomless black hole followed, a dark malady.
A thoughtless start to each day, except agony.
Deep depression and suicidal with life,
and a yearning to end it at forty-five.

A light at the end of the darkness at fifty.
Awards under my belt, I was moving on swiftly.

Here I am now at fifty-three,
healing the past, a new me.
Older wiser and stronger,
I'm a victim no longer.

Healing Myself and Finding My Purpose

This is my journey to wellness. It reads a bit like a "Who's Who" of illness, dis-ease and trauma and yet I know that for all the problems I have endured, most people have similar life stories in one way or another and there are many for whom life deals a much worse hand than mine. For this reason, I came to realise that if I can heal a "normal" lifetime of traumas then anyone can. So here it is, my life, my traumas and my journey back to wellness.

I was a child of the 1960s in England and throughout my childhood years, I succumbed to the usual common childhood illnesses; Measles, German Measles, Scarlatina, Mumps, Chickenpox, various ear infections and of course, multiple colds. I made a full recovery each time.

At the age of nine, I was sexually abused by a neighbour. Of course, I did not understand what happened, so I buried this deep inside me and kept it a secret from my family. It wasn't until much later when I was in my early twenties and after the birth of my son that I finally told my family. But after telling them, nothing changed in my life, I didn't heal the hurt and again, I covered up the memory.

When I was sixteen, I decided to leave home and live by myself. However, before I could make my way into the world, I was taken ill with Glandular Fever (caused by the Epstein Barr Virus). This not only affected my throat but also my joints, causing pain and weakness, keeping me at my mum's house longer. Overall, it was several weeks before I finally got back on my feet and moved out.

Once I was living on my own, an independent adult – albeit still a teenager, I developed eczema and reflux as a consequence of my newly found "carefree" lifestyle. Still being totally into the medical model, a quick visit to the doctor and I had some steroidal cream and antacid medications to relieve the symptoms. Partying resumed.

Later, around the age of nineteen and just after the untimely and very sad death of my stepfather, my weight ballooned as a result of developing Bulimia Nervosa. I would come home from work and proceed to binge eat, anything and everything, completely out of control. Then I would vomit it all back up again in total guilt. This was a daily "lifestyle" for me and I managed to put on around forty pounds. I subsequently dealt with it by not dealing with it, suppressing these emotions alongside the other now repressed emotions.

Then psoriasis appeared on both my now larger-than-ever thighs. One visit to my doctor later and I ended up with stronger steroidal cream than before. It was at some point during this outbreak that I began to wonder if I could heal the psoriasis myself... So, I spent the summer in shorts, getting the sun and sea air (living on the coast of Southern England) to my legs. It was a miracle: They healed!

Shortly after this, in my early twenties, I had my first child as a single parent. With this I found myself suffering from terrible post-natal depression. I was struggling on my own, my parenting skills were sorely lacking and I was frankly clueless. So, after a reluctant visit to the doctor, I ended up on prescription antidepressants for about the next year.

After a move back to the North of England for moral support, I met my husband-to-be and along came marriage. Talk about stress! But at least I was no longer coping on my own. With the newly found support in my husband, I healed the Bulimia Nervosa and stopped vomiting.

Then, in my late twenties, I started having low back pain without any physical trauma (I now realise this came from emotional trauma, after being sexually assaulted), diagnosed – at the time - as a bulging disc. Taking painkillers allowed me to continue working to bring in a much-needed income. Around the same time, I had a candida infection. I took medication after medication from the doctor then a gynaecologist, for two years, but the infection was not cured.

Absolutely fed up with taking so many pharmaceutical medications for so long and not healing, I decided to start taking control of my health. This was my turning point. I cut out all sugar and carbohydrates from my diet and healed the candida within a few months. I found a chiropractor who relieved the back pain through chiropractic manipulation.

What didn't help was having my car driven into from behind by a lorry while I was in it.

Anyway, around this time, we had another child, this time a daughter and a "joint venture" between myself and my husband. The birth was somewhat traumatic as I desperately wanted a home birth without painkillers but after several hours of screaming agony, the Midwife decided that discretion was the better part of valour and promptly packed me into an ambulance and off to the maternity unit where I eventually became the proud mother (and my husband the proud father) of our little girl. Now we were four.

Older, maybe a bit wiser and in my early thirties, we moved across the country as a result of my husband's job. With not knowing the area or anyone and two young children in tow, my husband at work all day, I went into a downward spiral back to depression. My skin became dry, my hair became thin, I was cold and tired all the time, I was putting on weight (again). I didn't want to go to the doctor, so just persevered. I now know I had an underactive thyroid.

A few years later we decided to try a new adventure and moved to the USA... This did not work out and nearly two years after heading west for a brighter better future, we headed back to the UK. I found a new job in the same hospital I had trained as a nurse and within months suffered from severe, debilitating headaches and a return of eczema. Not wanting to take any pharmaceuticals, I spent my days alternating between the sofa and our bed. After two weeks and a lot of family pressure, I finally went to my doctor. I was diagnosed with "stress" and prescribed strong painkillers. The doctor informed me these pain killers would damage my kidneys after six months of use! These kidney destroying tablets took the edge off the pain but didn't relieve it, so I decided a life of needing dialysis wasn't for me and stopped taking them.

I started researching what I could do to heal myself naturally and found a chiropractor who had published an article about the cause of my type of headache. He said it was related to the whiplash injury I had received in my car accident years ago. Six weeks later, with two treatments of manipulation a week, I was totally pain-free.

To heal my thyroid and eczema, I began supplementing with sea kelp for iodine, Brazil nuts for the selenium and vitamin D3. I also cleaned up my eating habits further, cutting out gluten and dairy and began making my own non-toxic cleaning, beauty and health products, following simple instructions from web pages. Within a couple of months, I felt like a different person, the eczema disappeared and I had much more energy.

Moving on and my mid-forties, I experienced some very troubling times at work and dark days that lasted almost three years, I finally hit rock bottom. Severely depressed, I drank alcohol in excess. It became impossible for me to work as I shut down and retreated into myself, finding it difficult to interact with people. I was lost, confused and desperate for it all to end. Unable to cope, every day became a battle for survival.

My family were concerned and tried many ways to reach me to help. I was so wrapped up in my grief and not receptive to their help. My blood pressure dropped from the normal, healthy 120/70 that it had been for years, to a very low, 80/40. My adrenal glands were now suffering from the severe stress I was under.

My lowest point came one evening in the kitchen, whilst ironing. Listening to my family laughing and joking in the lounge, I truly believed I was making their lives miserable and that they would be better off without me. I sobbed uncontrollably, inaudible to my family.

Although I wanted out, I was concerned about any mess I might leave for my family to deal with. In my mind, I went through multiple ways to end my life but couldn't imagine how I was going to do it; I was a coward and at the bottom of an abyss, without a way out.

A friend suggested that we go to the gym once a week and do two fitness classes, back-to-back. I thought that exercising would help me to feel better, so I agreed. I pushed myself hard in the classes. I was punishing myself and my body for the situation I found myself in.

One day, as I walked my dogs, all the sights and sounds around me came into my consciousness. I saw that the bare trees were now in bud, the sky was blue and harmonious birdsong filled the air. The cold easterly breeze blew through the trees, making them sway, the sky had turned from grey to blue and the sun shone between the clouds. I realised spring was on its way.

I was learning the art of mindfulness and was starting to feel a little better. There were days without tears and the abyss I was in still seemed vacuous but not quite so dark.

Meditation came next. I couldn't silence my negative mind-chatter so I started listening to guided meditations. I visualised the pictures they talked about. It brought me peace for the duration of the meditation. Slowly, over time, I tried different meditations; with my future in mind. I started to see and feel the future I wanted, where I was happy, at peace and successful.

I started practising gratitude. It was all about the little things; the weather was getting warmer, the love I had from my family, my friend taking me to the gym and I could sit without any negative mind chatter for a few minutes. I was grateful for all these things. My mood was lifting. I started to integrate back into life.

My tired adrenal glands made me crave salt. I added it to anything and everything, in great quantities, I couldn't get enough of it. Researching how to heal them, I started taking vitamin B complex supplements and ashwagandha. I made and used magnesium oil on my body, changed my cooking oil to coconut and increased my intake of avocados and green vegetables. Healing was slow and took several years but finally, my blood pressure is now a more normal reading.

After a move to Wales with my husband's promotion, in my late forties, I developed a frozen shoulder, right-sided. The pain was excruciating, keeping me awake at night. I found a local chiropractor and underwent treatment of manipulation with acupuncture and daily exercises. In less than three months, my shoulder was healed, without taking any pharmaceutical medications or resorting to surgery. Then my left shoulder became frozen…maybe out of sympathy with my right side? I returned to the chiropractor, had a repeat of treatment and healed that too.

As I turned fifty, I started having pain in my lower back, right hip and right knee, without any musculoskeletal trauma to initiate it. After all the research and healing I had done in previous years, I knew the cause of this was emotional pain. I acknowledged it was there, surrendered to it and meditated on the underlying cause. As I healed my fear of getting older and moving forwards in my life, I healed the pain.

After being sexually assaulted many years before by a person I trusted, I had suppressed the memory of it alongside the sexual abuse from my childhood that I also hadn't healed. It wasn't till I was in my fifties and doing a lot of inner healing, that I finally told my husband what had happened. Thankfully, he believed me and was very supportive.

Through further meditation, I realised that I was holding much resentment and anger for issues in my childhood as well as the sexual assault. I have since undertaken a lot of forgiveness work, for myself and those who hurt me, as well as let go of all the negative emotions I had towards myself and others. This took time and introspection but was worth it to be able to let go of so much.

I also realised that I firmly held onto some beliefs, passed on from key people in my younger years. I made active changes to the beliefs that no longer worked for me in the world I now live in and I found new strengths and coping abilities.

Finally, I truly understood the need to practise forgiveness, to forgive myself for not having the skills and knowledge to deal with the situations I found myself in throughout my life. I forgave others too, realising that we are all the product of our life experiences. This was truly liberating and I now understand how forgiveness, or the lack of it, plays a huge part in wellness and illness.

These days, I can honestly say, I am pain-free, with no headache, backache or joint ache. I have no thyroid or adrenal issues, no depression or low mood. My hair is much thicker and my skin is no longer dry or covered in eczema and psoriasis. Changing my lifestyle; food and drink choices, making my own non-toxic products, reducing stress, exercising and using some supplements for a while, has also played a part in my healing. I now understand that healing isn't just about improving our lifestyle, it is about loving ourselves enough to want to commit to healing.

In my role as a coach, I now assist others to heal themselves by helping them to assess their lives and find the root cause of their symptoms. I feel privileged to be alongside them on their healing journey, watching them grow and heal. I have found my purpose in life. It's not just to be a nurse to help others deal with their symptoms, it is as a coach, to empower others to heal themselves by finding the root cause of their symptoms.

Part Two - Healing Journeys of Extraordinary people

"Every human being is the author of his own health or disease"

Buddha

Allergies and Sensitivities

*"The soul always knows
what to do to heal itself.
The challenge is to silence
the mind"*

Caroline Myss

Chapter 1

Healing My Life-Threatening Allergies

As a child, I would constantly suffer from colds and coughs. I grew up in an environment where medicines were freely available as benefits where my father worked. When we fell sick, we would run to the 'pharmacy uncle' to get it ourselves. Calcium and vitamin C pills were tasty and a few of our favourites. Common cold medicines were too common. This went on for many years too. Over time antibiotics were my friends. They would manage my symptoms.

I got married in 2001. I had severe allergies, cold, cough, dust allergies, smoke sensitivity, symptoms that would change with the weather, becoming really severe and go on for almost a month if I did not medicate it. As these issues were so common, neither I nor anyone around me thought I had any major ailment. I have had bizarre rashes on my lips and other areas termed as candida and medicated. I had procedures done to check for worms and parasites too.

During my first pregnancy, I had two urine infections. My daughter was born in 2005, four weeks prematurely, whilst I had a urine infection.

While working in the USA, a colourful spread of berries, greens and fruit were a part of my diet, along with dairy. I was never a slim person but put on more weight. I suffered from fissures on and off.

In 2008, my second daughter was born and I suffered a severe cough during and after my caesarean. With this pregnancy, my constipation and fissures became very severe and I had to undergo a fissurectomy operation.

In 2010, on a coffee date with my husband, I ate puff pastries in a coffee shop. I had severe rashes the following day and my body became swollen. I got histamine shots to suppress those symptoms. They kept recurring with anything I ate – vegetables, fruits, biscuits, rice, there was no pattern. I had to take steroids for five days. If I did not take these, my extremities would become stone-like heavy. My throat would get swollen to even breathe or swallow saliva. An allergy specialist told me I had an auto-immune response and my body's immune system was confused, saying it would be a lifelong disease and medicines are my only hope.

By this time, I was desperate for a solution, I decided to look for an alternative and went for Ayurvedic treatment for a year which helped me reduce most of the severe symptoms like swelling and asphyxiation.

I decided to quit my medications, but then the allergies came back and this time with a vengeance. I was hospitalised twice between 2010-2012, barely able to move, literally sleeping all day as it would feel so painful and heavy. I tried homeopathy too without any new breakthroughs except that I found my tea was possibly causing my allergies and I quit milk-based tea. Being vegetarians in India, milk, yogurt, ghee is a staple food. I continued having ghee and milk in my coffee, curd was my favourite which continued too.

In 2012, one of my friends introduced me to an acupressure healer. It is here that I learned that the body will heal itself, provided we don't suppress the symptoms through medicines. All my allergies were actually my body's way of throwing out toxins. It was my true awakening. I felt foolish to have blindly believed in the power of medicines and having abused the body.

The healer told me that acupressure was just to aid the body and digestive rest was everything. I drank vegetable broth for many days, my nose ran like a tap for three to four months and my desperation towards medicines was quite severe. I had to de-addict my habits. I was asked to quit all medicines, including my steroids and it was extremely painful as I was so used to medicines. I did not have a habit of facing my symptoms. The healer gave me moral support.

I had to quit white poisons – dairy, refined flour and white sugar majorly. I would eat as per my body's call for hunger and thirst. Whenever my symptoms were really severe, I would only have vegetable broth. I was reassured that the eliminating (removal of toxic waste and recovery from ailments) will stop when my toxins had cleared. So, I continued my detox and waited.

My skin was affected by rashes all over. My mantra was vegetable broth. I included tender coconut water and lime water over time. As days turned to months, my cold, cough and allergies stopped. I was no longer gargling daily. My rashes became less painful, less severe, less frequent. With the new lifestyle, I also lost a lot of weight from 70 kgs to about 60 kgs.

I became a true plant-based vegan over the next few years, then I started helping my daughter heal from similar conditions. I learnt the power of raw, took nature cure classes and practiced natural lifestyle habits. I stopped visiting doctors in 2012.

In 2015, I had to take a hormonal tablet to stop my menstruation to observe a religious ritual after my father succumbed to cancer. Within ten to fifteen days, I suffered a severe elimination which resembled the chikungunya virus. I fasted on liquids and was in bed for a week without any side effects of joint pains. That was the day I stopped any form of pharmaceutical suppression even for any event.

By 2016, I leant the power of raw foods and started helping people heal based on my experiences. My spiritual journey also started during this year with learning chakra meditations. In 2017, I took nature cure classes that made my experience and knowledge structured.

I have now incorporated more raw foods into my lifestyle; I eat cooked food only once a day for dinner. I stay on liquids all morning, fruits for lunch and salad if I get hungry again, but I finish my oil-free, gluten-free, organic, whole food plant-based cooked dinner by 7pm.

The positives about this lifestyle are the amount of energy I have for the entire day; I can hit the gym on an empty stomach after only lemon water and my eliminations are much faster now I am on raw foods.

A very significant change I see is that I have experienced no crucial pains even when I have broken my bones. I had my wisdom tooth extracted where the surgeon used removable stitches and these stitches came off on their own after I healed on juicing and fruits. In all these cases, I did not take any medications. I used to juice fruits most of the days and ate fruits for about ten days.

Interestingly, many people have approached me to help them with their health issues including diabetes, hypertension, obesity, Lupus, allergies, reproductive issues, thyroid, hearing issues, autism and even cancer. I coach people about the body's innate wisdom to heal. I encourage them to take charge of their own health by making concrete changes in food and lifestyle.

The message I want to give people is that when making changes at home do not try to change anybody else. Many times, we end up in painful arguments and conflicting situations with family members. You have to respect their lifestyle choices. We have to motivate them through our own results. My husband and both my kids follow a plant-based healthy lifestyle today because I was patient and did not force anyone, but educated them as they saw the reflection in my own living habits. We do not visit doctors for healing. We visit them only when we need fixing of body parts.

Secondly, emotional and mental peace at home is very important. Bad food choices will keep you diseased for an entire lifetime, but may not kill you. But depression, energy loss through complex thinking and unresolved emotions can really cascade the effects of a bad lifestyle. This can actually manifest as cancer. Of course, our natural bodies will love a natural lifestyle, but it is extremely important that people find reasons to stay innately happy. Only emotional wellbeing can bring physical wellbeing. Natural living is a gift and an opportunity to help others with the same message we were gifted with. Be blessed.

Smitha Hemadri

Chapter 2

How I Healed Chemical and Electromagnetic Sensitivity

Back in the 80's I moved from New England to Boulder, Colorado and accepted a position at the University of Colorado as a secretary which required long hours sitting in front of a computer. The office setting had low ceilings with fluorescent lights and a small inadequately ventilated room with a large xerox copier. I worked in this setting for nine years and during that time I lived in three houses in various stages of remodeling — new carpet, paint and stain. At home, I also used an electric blanket on my bed. All were sources of environmental pollution, chemicals and electromagnetic fields, that I was exposed to over a long period of time.

After two years in my job, I began experiencing burning, stinging eyes and a focusing problem accompanied by various degrees of fatigue. As years passed, other seemingly unrelated symptoms developed: digestive disturbances, bladder pain and frequency of urination, hypoglycemia attacks, irregular heartbeat, sensitivities to pollens and food.

Finally, my chiropractor diagnosed me with two forms of environmental illness, electromagnetic sensitivity in 1993 and chemical sensitivity two years later.

What did I do to recover from this challenging illness?

The Doctor I chose to help me to heal was Sherry Rogers, an M.D. in Syracuse, NY who had environmental illness herself for sixteen years and recovered. Over three days I was tested for everything Dr Rogers considers an immune system stressor: Inhalant allergies, food allergies, candida in the digestive tract, nutritional deficiencies, hormonal imbalance, heavy metals. The seventh item on her list aside from the physical stressors was "stress". Dr Rogers calls her list the "total load" and insists that for a person to recover all immune system stressors need to be treated simultaneously.

I was positive for the first four items and she sent me home with her very comprehensive protocol which I followed to the letter for eighteen months, but I did not recover. While this was distressing at the time, it was a blessing in disguise as it forced me to look at the seventh item on Dr Rogers' list: *stress*. I estimate now that stress caused about eighty percent of my immune system weakness and the stress was emotional and spiritual in nature.

So, over the next several years it was necessary for me to examine my inner workings, and I did this at a place called the Option Institute in the Berkshires of western Massachusetts. Institute mentors offer adult programs on happiness (and illness is considered a form of unhappiness) helping people to discover the beliefs behind situations in their life that aren't working and causing varying degrees of unhappiness. I was assisted to closely examine the "emotional stressors" that contributed to the demise of my immune system and, most importantly, the beliefs that were behind them.

By emotional stressors I mean fear-based emotions such as anger, bitterness, envy, jealousy, worry, anxiety, etc., also fear-based emotional ways of reacting to life; feeling rejected or abandoned, feeling guilty, judgment of self or others, etc.

Here are my personal emotional stressors which I had to address to lessen the load on my immune system in order to recover:

Feelings of rejection
Feelings of guilt
Wanting/needing to be perfect
Making myself responsible for other people's happiness and unhappiness
Living my life from a "should" or "have to" standpoint
Difficulty in asking for what I wanted or needed

In effect, these were all ways I didn't love myself.

How did this come about? Where did I learn all these ways of reacting fearfully in my world? Not surprisingly in childhood.

It began with a belief formed in my early years that I was not loved by my mother and continued on in a way that did not serve me when I copied errant behaviors which were modeled by a number of key adults I loved or respected. The unfortunate result was a child who grew into adulthood with low self-esteem and self-worth, feelings that can have a very negative effect on immune system strength if not released before they become embedded.

I spent a total of two and a half years at the Option Institute, in programs to discover and release many beliefs and ways of being that were contributing to the demise of my immune system. During this time, I also studied and became a mentor with the purpose of assisting others as Institute mentors had helped me.

When I returned home to Colorado from the Option Institute my health was the best it had ever been and I believed myself to be past my most challenging sensitivities and I was ready to resume a "normal" life. If any emotional stressors manifested, I reasoned, I had "tools" to apply before my immune system was negatively impacted. But, alas, what I was not aware of were the beliefs I hadn't uncovered at the Institute; still operating under the surface, these beliefs and ways of living life needed to be brought to light and released before my healing could be complete.

One fateful day the sensitivities resurfaced with a vengeance and this time, I had learned enough to suspect the root cause of the latest downturn. The stressor was spiritual in nature and I made plans to visit a world-famous healing center to seek help to address it.

Due to my religious upbringing as a child, my relationship with a Higher Power left a lot to be desired. A major issue that came to the surface at the healing center was the realization that while I knew at an intellectual level that I was loved by this one I called God, I could not feel that love in my heart. I was assisted to remedy this difficulty in an awe-inspiring way which I've recounted for those interested in my second book entitled "Coming Home to Love".

Other spiritual issues I became aware of during multiple trips to this same healing center:

Lack of trust in Source
The necessity of asking for what I want in life
The ramifications of judgment, both of myself and others
Letting go of the need to control
Healing power of forgiveness of both myself and others

I was helped to see how all these issues were fear-based, more ways I was separated from Love, love for both the Divine as well as myself.

I am happy to tell you that after my fourth trip to this beautiful healing center I came home free of the sensitivities I had suffered to environmental pollution. The first positive sign of this after returning home was the ability to put gas in my own car without reaction, a simple task that I had been unable to do for many years.

While my physical healing was complete, I continued to observe my thoughts and behavior patterns and made a solid effort to improve my relationship with this One I call the Divine. In current days I have been blessed to find a very powerful and effective spiritual path which I lovingly follow and intend to continue for the remainder of my earthly life.

Marcia Murphy

Author of

"Healing Environmental Illness from Within" (available on Amazon)
"Coming Home to Love" (available from me)

Also working on a third book which will combine the two books above to tell the complete story in one volume. I don't know how long that will take to finish, but I am hopeful for some time this year.

Asthma, Eczema, Autism

"Healing is not an overnight process, it is a daily cleansing of pain, it is a daily healing of your life"

Leon Brown

Chapter 3

Healing Asthma with Naturopathy

For as long as I could remember I had a cough, not just a little tickle but a cough that made people stare and move away from me on the train, a cough that got me kicked out of sleepovers and a cough that at times would make me throw up as well as keep me awake for hours at night. I'd get it about three times a year and it would last anywhere from four to eight weeks and at times I felt like it was permanently there.

After fifteen years of seeing my doctor, I was finally diagnosed with Cough Variant Asthma. I was informed to use an inhaler morning and night and any time I felt the cough coming on, to start taking antibiotics, which were put on a repeat prescription. I wasn't happy with this, at twenty-eight years old how could I be on lifelong medication? I was starting to become aware of the damaging effects of the antibiotics and knew I just couldn't live my life like this.

I found a lovely naturopath called Jess. At my first consultation, I offloaded all of my symptoms including the acne around my chin, which developed into a boil that lasted over two weeks, after eating dairy, as well as experiencing diarrhoea. She listened sympathetically as I cried about how awful I felt. I now refer to her as my angel, although she always tells me that I did all the work. Over a period of three months, I saw Jess six times, once every two weeks. She was a kinesiologist and used to ask my body what was the main concern of the session.

She suggested that I made changes to my diet and I started introducing juices and smoothies. Every morning I made and drank a large glass of celery juice, then thirty minutes later I had a smoothie consisting of a handful of blueberries, a medjool date, banana, plant-based milks, spinach, flax seeds and chia seeds. I also started to say affirmations; 'I am healthy, happy and fantastic', throughout the day (something that I still do now!) I would have a salad with rocket and quinoa, tomatoes, avocado and olive oil, salt and pepper for lunch and dinner would be something gluten-free and vegetable based such as curry and brown rice.

I took supplements of slippery elm and zinc as well as homeopathy pills. Once every two weeks, I would take five tablespoons of castor oil before bed for a natural colonic. As the weeks went on, I started doing twenty-four hour fruit only fasts, followed by a water-only fast for twenty-four hours.

I started sleeping through the night and waking up feeling refreshed. I then did a five day water only fast. I found it incredibly difficult, having never done one before, but on day three, I noticed my hearing improve (which is not something I thought needed improving) and on day five, I broke my fast with a smoothie which tasted amazing.

Finally, I did a parasite cleanse which I think was crucial to my healing. I ate only fruit for five days straight whilst taking magnesium oxygen pills, which flushed out my system and I took clove and wormwood tinctures. On day three, I passed a parasite that was about two centimetres long. I immediately felt like a weight had been lifted from my shoulders.

After three months of working with Jess, I was at an optimal weight, my skin had completely cleared, I could eat dairy again with no side effects and my cough was gone.

It's now been a year and a half since I completed my body cleanse and my cough is still absent. My doctor rang me just to check in and see how I was doing. I told him that I had healed my asthma through changing my diet and the use of fasting, he was very impressed. Maybe one day doctors might give advice might be similar to that of my naturopath, but until then individual health is very much down to the individual.

Sadly, I think there are too many conflicts of interests for the healthcare system to ever really change but I hope my story helps someone improve their health. There is a light at the end of the tunnel if you are willing to see it through different eyes.

Since my healing, I am training to become a naturopath, studying naturopathic nutrition and kinesiology. It has great success in healing many illnesses which sadly, many doctors believe are incurable and lifelong.

Alice Taylor

Chapter 4

Acceptance of Asthma

As a kid, I was highly active in sports. My passions were soccer and basketball. I played soccer for longer, in fact, I played till I was nineteen. From the age of six years old till around my late twenties, I suffered from asthma.

Sometimes after games, my inhaler would run out of steroids and my parents would have to race me to the emergency as I was wheezing and couldn't breathe. My Dad who was an alpha male couldn't see me get a shot, so he would wait outside the doctor's office as the nurse and doctor held me down to give me my shot, which felt like a nail going into my arm. It hurt. Really hurt.

The asthma would linger after the age of nineteen and would come back at interesting times. Mostly I observed in times of stress. One day I caught myself being overly critical of myself, and felt my lungs constrict and body tighten. Then the shortness of breath, and wheezing.

It was the first time I caught what might be going on with my asthma. I had grown up with it and never knew there was a way out.

So, I decided to implement something. When I felt the lungs constrict and heard the critical voice in my head; rather than judge it or condemn or say, "Why is this happening to me?", instead I would allow and observe. This became magical because as I observed the stress and criticism, it allowed for more air to fill up my lungs. Then I could focus on what we call now "conscious breathing".

I continued this process and before I knew it, the asthma was gone. I haven't experienced it now for twenty years.

I continued to use this method with sensations or aches or pain in my body. By accepting what was happening, observe it without judgement or condemnation, and breathe. It has helped me in loving myself by first accepting what is unfolding now inside. And so, when I deal with unruly people around me, the attention is always within, and checking in with my inner self on what is coming up.

How great to see why asthma entered my life. It was my biggest teacher and helped me to learn to accept myself no matter what. What a great gift.

David Matthew Brown

David Matthew Brown is a Shaman, who uses energy, breathwork, counselling, intuition, and clairaudience to work with clients. He has given over six hundred and fifty talks around the globe, is a published author, Dad, and has coached over three hundred girls and teens in soccer.

Chapter 5

Healing Eczema Through Overhauling My Lifestyle

My journey started as a child with the skin condition, eczema. I had a severe reaction mainly on the backs of my legs, my arms and my neck. I felt embarrassed and self-conscious whenever those unsightly red marks and scaly skin were on display. It was very itchy and uncomfortable at times. I found some soothing relief from available, over-the-counter emollient creams, calamine lotions and bath oils.

The cause of the eczema was unclear and I was never tested to find out the origins. I felt that it may have been due to an allergy or intolerance of some kind; possibly to dairy products or a sensitivity to one or more chemicals. To help manage my symptoms, we made changes to some of our washing routines and processes e.g. washing our clothes with "washing balls" which don't typically use detergent or using more "sensitive" body care products.

Many kids grow out of eczema; however, I continued to have it into my teenage years and my twenties. It was aggravated by hot weather and during periods of extreme stress and unhealthy diet lapses. I decided to visit my doctor for some professional assistance and was prescribed the standard steroid hydrocortisone cream. I do not recall being given advice on what might be causing it or being referred to a dermatologist. I applied the steroid cream in the more severe cases and it did help to clear up my skin for many years.

However, I wanted a more permanent solution, preferably a more natural one, and to not be reliant on pharmaceutical lotions and potions. I also started to have concerns about possible side effects from the prolonged use of steroid creams so used them sparingly, in addition to the emollient creams.

At that time, I was also using conventional sun protection lotions. I always opted for sun protection creams for "sensitive skin" with the highest protection possible. However, reading the ingredients of some popular brands of sun protection creams which claim to be for "sensitive skin", I found that many contain aluminium derivatives and all manner of unpronounceable chemicals. My suspicions are that my skin may have adversely reacted to some of the chemicals contained in these products.

It was once I hit my thirties that I started to take more of an active interest in natural health and alternative remedies. I was more mindful of any synthetic preservatives or additives contained in these pharmaceutical products. Even if the quantities were small, there was the possibility that they could be toxic with prolonged use or cause side effects. I researched the list of ingredients on the information leaflet. Interestingly, two of the possible side effects of the calamine lotion product claiming to help heal rashes and itchy skin are indeed rashes and itchy skin. Thankfully, I found plenty of natural, homemade calamine lotion recipes online, which are a better alternative and kinder to the body long term.

So, in the last ten years, I have gone on quite a crusade to radically overhaul my lifestyle, my diet and my skincare and cleaning regimes. I have avidly researched how I can use self-healing techniques and natural products as much as possible in preference to conventional medical solutions. I will share with you some of the factors which have helped me not only to heal my eczema which has very rarely made an appearance in recent years (only in extreme stress and diet lapses!) but also changed my life both mentally and physically for the better.

1. I favour a diet low in refined sugar, refined carbohydrates and processed foods; and high in fruits, vegetables, nuts, seeds, healthy fats, whole grains and more natural unrefined sweeteners.
2. I practise intermittent fasting almost daily which is believed to help reduce inflammation and maintain a healthy weight.
3. I choose natural remedies for colds and coughs e.g., lemon, Echinacea, ginger, garlic etc. I understand that my body's best

form of defence is the natural immune system which is also enhanced with good sleep, exercise, a healthy diet and managed stress levels.

4. I regularly take vitamin and mineral supplements, such as Vitamin C, Zinc, B complex and Magnesium.
5. For sun protection, I seek shade and cover up when required and occasionally use a natural sun protection product e.g., containing Aloe Vera, zinc oxide, coconut oil and lovely essential oils. I feel happier allowing my body access to more sunshine and Vitamin D.
6. I have replaced all my synthetic creams, shampoos, soaps, deodorants, toothpastes etc with more natural alternatives. My deodorants and moisturiser are now homemade and I am experimenting with making more products.
7. I use homemade cleaners containing white vinegar, bicarbonate of soda etc. They are very cheap to make and they work well believe me. I limit my use of other chemical products or use more natural alternatives.
8. I completely stopped using emollient and steroid creams and switched to natural moisturisers such as coconut oil, aloe vera, shea butter etc. Although for me good hydration and a healthy diet equate to good skin.
9. I changed my lifestyle and living circumstances which included moving from an urban to a rural location and living a more small-scale and back to nature style of living.
10. I relaxed my working life and started working part-time more. This created more time for sleep, outdoor pursuits and engaging in my favourite pastimes.

Now it could have been a combination of some or all of these factors which contributed to healing my eczema, improving my overall health and wellbeing, and also helping me to lose weight. Although being human, I still have the occasional indulgence.

My self-healing journey has included hours of self-learning, research and watching documentaries. However, if this is not for you, there are many natural health professionals i.e. naturopaths, homeopaths, nutritionists etc who can help guide you and support you along this empowering and enlightening journey which can help to change your life.

All these experiences inspired me to create my own platform "Simple Balance Today", to help others on their journey.

Susie Berns

Chapter 6

Healing Myself Through Healing My Son

My healing journey extends into generations ahead and behind me. I knew early in adulthood I'd be the one to impact my family. The majority of the healing I needed was spiritual and emotional.

Always having a rather robust constitution, many of the physical illnesses I experienced were easy to resolve with changing habits- not smoking, not eating processed food, not drinking to excess. I learned a lot about the body and gained much practical knowledge through my training and practice of massage therapy. Adopting a yogic lifestyle did worlds of good for me and I believe was the key to my genetic expression glow up. My family members were not as fortunate.

My father was a lifelong drinker and smoker so all health issues he had were easy to correlate. My mother was not as easy to figure out. She neither drank nor smoked but she regularly got rather serious illnesses or dire events and overcame them, so much that I saw that no diagnosis was permanent or impossible to overcome. Lyme disease, migraines, Multiple Sclerosis, Trans Ischaemic Attacks (TIA's), allergies, she had them all and never did she let them beat her. She was my inspiration and model in healing. However, the one thing she never addressed or could resolve was her emotional trauma and this would be the obstacle that prevented her being here today. So many of the symptoms and illnesses pointed to MTHFR gene mutation but I was not to learn about that until after she had passed over from colon cancer.

Although my second son was born at home naturally and given no vaccines, after about one year old he began some peculiar behaviors and lost the few words he had started using. I couldn't understand what I was seeing and no one suggested autism to me but that was what I suspected, so I began my research.

When I asked my acupuncturist friend about speech delays and distortions, she asked if he was tongue-tied. The answer is yes, though he was exclusively breastfed and had no issue with latch, I could see that little heart shape at the tip of his tongue. This led me to midline defects which led to MTHFR mutations which was the missing piece, for him and my mother. Instantly I could understand every symptom on both sides of my family for generations. I did not wait for genetic testing to confirm what I knew. I prayed for guidance to set me on a path to healing my son.

At age two he was nonverbal, non-interactive, very little eye contact or receptive language shown, moderate to bad eczema flares, stimulation seeking, and not potty trained. My intuition said a hard no to interventions and therapies. I knew from my research into MTHFR that toxicity was a factor and the inflammation was causing much of the symptoms I saw. I continued my fervent pleas to God for the way and soon in the Facebook groups I was in, I saw mention of a zeolite spray called TRS. It was almost as if there was an aura around these posts, a highlight or subtle attraction for me to read them. I knew this was the answer to my prayers. I joined more groups, placed my order and waited for my bottles to arrive.

While I waited, I researched more. I trusted the answer I was given yet I wanted to understand and have confidence in what I was doing. I understood perfectly the function of the mineral and I knew how to support the body from my years of experience prior.

I started the sprays on myself just to be sure all was as it seemed and a week later, I started the rest of my family. Within forty-eight hours the majority of his eczema was gone, and in the second week, he began to say his a,b,c's. His language slowly bloomed and behaviors improved over the following months with spurts in development following each wave of candida die-off. Nothing will compare to hearing "I love you, mom" when less than a year prior I wondered if there would ever be any words. Detoxification was the answer to begin his healing.

After two and a half years, I was ready to try something more to support him. My friend who is a gifted energy worker suggested Emotion Code therapy. We began clearing his trapped emotions and he really began to bloom again. We began to work on his quantum DNA, and I was guided to ask for healing his gut biome. It was several weeks of work and I can tell you it was so worth it because now this child is fully conversational as of this month. Many sensory issues are now resolved and the gains keep coming. I am thrilled beyond belief that my five-year old son may soon be fully recovered from the spectrum. Even if he retains some behaviors it matters not to me. All I want for him is to be as healthy and happy as possible, and now I see him thriving instead of surviving.

You may wonder how this is my healing story. Of course, I've benefitted from detoxing myself also. I had no idea how many symptoms I had were tied to liver issues, candida and parasites that are now gone. Lifelong things I lived with like dry skin, dandruff, cracked heels, bloated belly, keratosis pilaris, a fatty lipoma, sun spots on my cheeks... all gone now when I had thought they were just normal aging mommy issues!

But more than that, the horrible guilt I had for what I perceived as failing my mother and then my son was resolved. I blamed myself for not knowing the difference between folic acid and folate, listening to what was meant to be helpful guidance to take more folic acid during pregnancy when really that was likely what triggered the genetic expression to cripple the detoxing ability of my child.

I shamed myself for not figuring out what the sacral dimple meant when I had seen it on my mother and my son. Why had I not known? Well, epigenetics was no field of mine nor was it even common chat amongst natural health practitioners at that time. It's easy to say that it's not my fault but certainly I felt it was and even more so my job to figure out how to recover and heal my child.

I have succeeded, and I share my experiences with others to detox and support their families in this healing journey. This has healed my spirit and my heart along with my family. Resolving the emotional and spiritual distress has improved my internal stress levels which certainly will help my bodily systems in the big picture. We will all move forward with gratitude and mindfulness, enjoying each day, and I know my mother in heaven is proud of me for solving some of the puzzles of our ancestors for the good of our future.

Grace Hughes

Autoimmune Disorders

"Let Food Be Thy Medicine and Medicine Be Thy Food"

Hippocrates

Chapter 7

How to Survive Without Gluten and Restore Your Health from Celiac Disease or Gluten Sensitivity

---

I'm far from healed. Saying I'm healed assumes there is an end point to this journey. I accept that I'll always be in the process of healing. In fact, there is no such thing as being "healed" when you have celiac disease.

Celiac disease is a rare autoimmune disease that affects 1 in 100 people. This disease is triggered every time I eat a tiny protein called gluten. Gluten is found in products that contain wheat, barley or rye, and derivatives of these grains.

Gluten seems like a harmless food, and it's an essential and necessary ingredient in giving bread its stretchy, doughy appeal. I had no idea that with every bite of pizza, bread or pasta I took, I was contributing to the decline and eventual destruction of my small intestine. The small intestine is an essential organ charged with absorbing and distributing nutrients from the food you eat to every organ and cell in your body. Without a functioning small intestine, and subsequent distribution of essential nutrients throughout your body, your body can't function properly and disease ensues.

Before I learned I had celiac disease, I began to suffer from daily painful bloating, embarrassing gas, nutrient depravity, and chronic fatigue. I had no idea gluten was behind it all until one day, after complaining to my doctor, she suggested we run some blood "tests."

Who knew this innocent protein that I loved for thirty-four years of my life could be used to create chemical warfare in my body... but that's exactly what it was doing.

In a quest to heal my body, I had no choice but to implement a strict, gluten-free diet. In doing so, I had to ignore the nay-sayers, the people who dismissed my diet as a fad, and those would didn't believe it was possible that the tiny gluten protein could be the source of all my health woes.

While ditching gluten relieved many of my painful and annoying symptoms over time, it wasn't the cure-all "diet" it promised to be. I only felt marginally better. It turns out I had removed the irritant making and keeping me sick (gluten), but I had done little to address the damage left behind in gluten's wake.

After eating gluten-free for a full year, and still feeling semi-lousy at the end of each day, I had a realization that there is more to the gluten-free diet than meets the eye. Sure, I had removed the irritating protein that got me into this mess in the first place, but I hadn't nurtured the deep wounds left behind in my body.

It is upon this realization that the start of my healing journey would truly begin. This journey started the day I *woke up*, so to speak, not the day I was diagnosed.

I began to realize – and truly understand – that food could either hurt or heal me. I realized that trading wheat donuts for gluten-free donuts wasn't actively contributing to healing the wounds inside me, and it was quite possibly further damaging my body.

I began to study gluten disorders and nutrition in earnest. I enrolled in the Institute for Integrative Nutrition to learn how I could heal my body. I began to fully understand the importance of food as medicine (based on the famous quote once said by Hippocrates, the father of modern medicine). I studied gluten disorders in earnest. And I had an epiphany that I had been *doing food* all wrong my entire life.

To heal my body, which I actively do every day, I began to employ the following tactics:

Eating the Right Foods: I learned that the gluten-free diet isn't just about swapping pizza for gluten-free pizza; rather, it's an opportunity to change your entire diet for the better. To counteract the nutrient depravity I experienced for years, I work hard to load up on anti-inflammatory foods every day – including plenty of fruits and vegetables – so I can nourish every cell in my body. Whereas I rarely ate vegetables in my pre-celiac years, today I eat them with every meal.

Being Strict: Even a crumb of gluten could set back my health for weeks, so I'm certain to follow the gluten-free diet to a T. I don't do it half-heartedly or when it's convenient. I never eat gluten. No exceptions.

Resting the Digestive System: I never thought about how hard my body had to work to digest all the food I ate until my diagnosis. Today, however, I make a conscious effort to rest my digestive system between meals (no snacking), and I stop eating after 7pm every evening to allow my body a full twelve hours to rest and digest each night. I drink cold-pressed green juices regularly, which not only flood my body with vital nutrients but also makes those nutrients readily absorbable by my body without making my digestive system work one bit.

Limiting Sugar: Not only did I had to end my love affair with gluten, but I had to take a hard look at my relationship with sugar. I loved all things sweet, and I needed to tame my sweet tooth before it got the best of me. Limiting sugar, combined with a good probiotic, restored balance in my belly and helped me feel my best, healthy self.

Changing My Mindset: I once saw celiac disease, and the subsequent gluten-free diet, as a burden or curse in my life. Today, however, I see celiac disease as a true gift, a blessing. Celiac disease was a course correction for me, putting me on a path towards good health and potentially saving my life. Today I have the mindset of a healthy person, not a sick person.

Celiac disease will always be a part of me, and for the foreseeable future, the only way to treat this disease is by changing how I eat. I'm grateful that I can manage it through the food on my plate; and I realize that every time I eat a healthy, g-free meal, I'm voting for good health one gluten-free forkful at a time.

Jenny Levine Finke

Certified Integrative Nutrition Coach

Author of

Dear Gluten, It's Not Me, It's You: How to Survive Without Gluten and Restore Your Health from Celiac Disease or Gluten Sensitivity

Jenny lives in Denver, Colorado with her husband, their two kids, and their rescue dog, Buddy. When she's not blogging, she's cooking up a storm in the kitchen, listening to books while walking her dog, or spending quality time with her family.

Chapter 8

Open-Minded About Healing

Until the point of becoming unwell, I had a healthy active lifestyle. I was training regularly at the gym, cycling, walking my dogs for miles, regularly attending dance classes and I learnt the trapeze. I was a very social person, always up for a night out. Life was to be grabbed and shaken with both hands.

When my symptoms started, I thought they were just the general aches and pains to be expected at my time of life, just over forty. The aches and pains became worse. Standing was painful and movement, in general, was stiff and painful.

In January 2014, I woke with a headache that lasted several months! I became light and sound sensitive and my vision became blurred at times. When all three occurred together, I was overwhelmed and disorientated.

Once I found a doctor who would take me seriously, I was referred to Rheumatology. In the meantime, I was treated for Fibromyalgia or Myalgic Encephalomyelitis (ME) with various medications and signed off work for a month.

I managed to go back to work for two weeks before being signed off again. This went against my work ethic but was a necessary intervention by my doctor. My employer became remote and at times hostile. I tried everything I could to engage with them, but their behaviour was both surprising and questionable.

My doctor referred me for various scans and numerous blood tests, which all returned as normal. I was prescribed a plethora of medication and ended up taking forty tablets a day and wearing a Fentanyl patch for years. These medications did not help resolve my symptoms or improve my health. I lost the ability to talk and started having mini seizures. At one point, I was tested for a stroke.

Thankfully, all was clear. My Doctor and Pain Management Consultant changed my medication and it became apparent I had a reaction to Gabapentin!

I was finally diagnosed with Fibromyalgia and ME in August 2014. It was a bittersweet day. The relief I was not going mad was soon surpassed by the fear of this potentially being the rest of my life. I was psychologically struggling with unwelcome changes in my life, leaving me depressed and anxious, not able to leave the house and unable to walk without being in burning pain. I was not able to drive, dress, wash, shower, shave, prepare food in the normal way, or do anything normally.

My lowest point came when I received a letter of dismissal from my employer and at the same time, I became registered as disabled. I am ashamed to say I no longer wanted to be part of this world. Luckily, at this time, my partner was with me. We spent many hours talking and I finally saw sense.

The pain and fatigue became so severe at times that I was unable to get out of bed for days. The pain was relentless, from the soles of my feet to the top of my head. Wearing clothes was painful too; socks hurt my ankles and waistbands on trousers hurt my abdomen.

The duvet was too heavy and would increase the pain I was already in, meaning that sleep was out of the question at times. I could be awake for forty-eight hours, sleep for a few hours and up again for forty-eight hours. Eventually, my body would give up and I would sleep for eighteen hours, then wake up in excruciating pain. The cycle would then start all over again.

I attended a ten-week pain management course, it didn't help. I tried Chiropractors, Acupuncture, Physiotherapy, meditation, self-help books, relaxation techniques and a whole host of things. Nothing worked.

I was invited to try a new treatment called Physiokey. My first treatment was on the 16th of February 2016. I was not holding my breath for anything to happen. How wrong could I have been?

When I arrived for my appointment, I was unable to walk more than five meters with crutches. After two days of intense Physiokey treatments, I walked away without crutches and I was able to walk up a flight of stairs. It was amazing. When I got home my partner was shocked and said, "it's lovely to meet you again".

More treatments followed over a period of months. With each treatment, I felt better, physically, emotionally, mentally. Because of my health improvement, I decided to stop all the prescribed medications. Within six weeks, I was off all of the forty daily tablets and the Fentanyl patches prescribed by my Doctor.

I had an opportunity to study and become a Physiokey therapist. I grabbed it with both hands. I was motivated and met the challenge head-on. While having treatments I was skilfully being put through the training and understanding of the Physiokey device.

I studied Anatomy and Physiology which is a criterion of becoming a practitioner. Eventually, I passed all my exams and started working with real patients, people like me who endured years of pain, medications, test and so on. Now several years on I still can't quite believe the massive journey, through the bowels of hell and coming to a place where I can help myself and others.

I still have Fibro and ME which I self-manage with Physiokey treatments. Day to day life is as normal as I can make it, with an eighty-five to ninety percent reduction in pain, fatigue and depression. Being able to treat myself if I have a flare-up or feel it is necessary, is wonderful.

Taking ownership and responsibility for my own health and well-being has created a huge shift in my willingness to throw tablets down my throat without questioning. My Doctor was wonderful, but I realise now the answers are not with him, they are with me. I still do not take any pharmaceutical medications.

I love helping other people to heal themselves, as I have. My business Arc Wellbeing is going from strength to strength. Patients trust that I know what they are feeling, the pain, isolation, desperation and sheer gravity of grieving for the loss of your old self.

The journey is not over. Treating myself has allowed me to push my boundaries and I have recently completed a thirty-day self-imposed Movement/Fitness challenge. I am driven to keep finding new ways to help myself and build strength, stamina and endurance. I have not found a cure, but I have found an effective way to self-heal.

Would I change the fact I have Fibro and ME? NO, I would go through it all again. I have learnt so much about myself, worked on my resolve and tenacity, found a wonderful way to self-heal and more importantly and far more rewarding for my soul, is to be able to help others.

Paul Dumper

Chapter 9

Healing Is Aligning

I am writing to you from a gorgeous villa in Bali, with a beautiful pool that overlooks the Balinese rice fields. Tomorrow I am moving to a Tarzan Tree House in the middle of the jungle! I moved to Bali from the UK in November 2020 despite seemingly "limiting" circumstances. I was also in full-time work that, although I was good at, it was not in ALIGNMENT with my real gifts and soul mission, which is to dismantle the establishment that says we cannot heal, bring healing women together, reawaken the Wild Woman within and heal ourselves so we can heal the planet.

The last flare I had was January 2020. Ten months earlier, I was living in the Canary Islands, beautiful but, where were my Wild Women? I had a quiet life, I taught English, I went out with ex-pats at the weekend to get drunk, then I got bored with that and rarely left my house.

I had been suffering from symptoms since 2010 and diagnosed around 2014 with multiple chronic illnesses including Fibromyalgia Syndrome, Chronic Fatigue, Irritable Bowel, Anxiety and Depression and then there were all the ones not formally diagnosed but just sort of 'noted'; Carpal Tunnel, Chronic Migraines, pain with intercourse, painful menstruation, hives, temporomandibular joints syndrome (TMJ), asthma, recurring infections like sinusitis, ear infections, tonsillitis, urine infections (UTIs), then there was the Insomnia, Postural Orthostatic Tachycardia Syndrome (POTS), constant nausea, and then the pain; constant back pain, restless leg syndrome, sciatica, neck pain, arm pain, costochondritis, stomach pain - heartburn, and the bloating. It isn't really important what I "had". This is not a manual for healing specific diagnoses.

My stance is that we're all healing the same inner wounds. These repressed, unhealed, forgotten, ignored and shameful wounds we carry within us that can physically manifest as this or that diagnosis; and sure, there is the symbolism of the symptom, what it represents- i.e. if it is burning, pinching, suffocating, draining, too much, not enough, etc, it gives us a pretty good reflection of where in OUR LIFE we are burning or draining ourselves. Then there is the body-mind link. We form our own body around our mind. We form our posture by how we feel about ourselves. We form ourselves on the physical, cellular level, and in my own healing, the first thing I did was to be willing to accept that on some level I created illness. Yes. I needed to take all responsibility for the creation of all those two hundred plus symptoms, in order to step out of my own perception of being a victim and overhaul my life.

Not everyone is ready to hear this Truth. I wasn't when I was diagnosed and I suffered for about ten years- from sixteen years old to twenty-six years old. The first half of being twenty-six, I was sick and depressed, in the second half, I healed myself.

Now that I knew I had created all this illness; it was my duty to figure out WHY. I did this by cultivating an intuition practice with myself, with the depths of my Self. I learnt how to reconnect to my body and reframe my old, outdated beliefs about my body "attacking me", working "against me", "hates me" and whatever other victim language I was choosing to keep myself small and defenceless. I accepted that in every moment my body is healing me. It still is now, of course, I no longer have any chronic illnesses, no chronic symptoms whatsoever, but my body is forever healing. Isn't that exactly what life is? It's healing ourselves on every single level. This is beyond diet changes, and taking a certain supplement my love. I needed to look at who I was, where was my passion? What was my karmic service to this Earth on this timeline? Who needs to be forgiven? What do I need to do to continue to let myself evolve?

The physical illnesses? They heal as a side-effect.   I'm serious.

If you are expecting to heal your body with some changes here and there but continue to surround yourself with toxic people who walk all over you, a toxic job you hate or that drains you, a life situation you find limiting, controlling or just BORING, if you continue to play the victim in areas of your life, if you continue to block yourself from receiving love, miracles and abundance, if you keep your consciousness stifled and asleep with mundanity, criticism, judgement, gossip, stubbornness, fears and resentments; you are missing the whole point of your healing journey.

Healing is a spiritual practice.

Healing happened when I did the thing I was afraid to do for the longest time. Healing happened when I decided I was already worthy and then navigated my life around that core belief. Life mirrors back to us exactly what we feel, what we say we want, and what we think we deserve. On some level when I was sick, I believed I was a sick girl, with all these old poor me traumas of what other people did to me. I believed that I couldn't have what I wanted because that's how life is, and I believed I did not deserve things like ease, peace, health or pleasure, because I believed they didn't exist for me, or that they only came with tremendous struggling or that I have to "earn it" by being "good" and when I'm "bad", there will be consequences/punishments i.e. chronic, debilitating symptoms.

I left Spain when I finally accepted it wasn't my end destination on my journey in healing. My partner of three years dumped me, which I have now accepted and can see all the ways that being together kept me being sick (although we loved each other, the love was limiting both of us). I made the conscious decision to heal and that I am a healer, which asked of me to fearlessly create my own coaching business for women who heal and show UP for themselves.

I dropped all sense of poor me victim patterns. I dropped all the assumptions and limitations I had made up in my head about my capabilities and what is possible for me and in this world. Yes, I made real changes to ALIGN with my life as a healed woman. These were not sacrifices. I am vegan because I no longer subscribe to the meat and dairy industry; when I was sick, I didn't care about animals, the agenda or myself. But when a woman in healing wakes up to the fact she has been played by a global industry that profits when she is a customer of healthcare, that Wild Woman never goes back to sleep again.

What else did I change? I already had my yoga practice and other ways to connect and love myself. When I healed, I decided these were no longer things I had to "muster up energy" for. I do these things with love because I love myself. I changed some routines because again, sleeping in until eleven or noon was another way for me to not love myself and get in my own way because then I'd complain of being drowsy and "not having enough time". Even though it is ME who creates my perception of time. I also choose to be a non-drinker and non-smoker after eight years of binging and chain-smoking.

These are not sacrifices, and these are not in themselves, "the cure". They were ways for me to hate myself, and hating myself is a limitation to my radical healing. I have worked courageously and with determination on my energy field and who I attract in; now I radically love myself, I am not on the same bandwidth anymore with people who abuse me in any way. I choose to align myself with receiving miracles in the form of people, things, experiences; and that's what my whole life is every single day.

My body is my best friend in this whole Universe. My body chose me for this particular simulation of life and it's my duty to love and honour this temple.

My mind is my wise mother-figure that guides me. It is from our mind that we manifest EVERYTHING.
My soul is the same energy as yours and we're all running around this matrix game forgetting we are all droplets of the same powerful force. Then we heal ourselves and remember who we are.

Unleash yourself, sister, from everything and anything that does not serve you in stepping up and out, LOUD and proud, as the You, you really are. You are not chronic diagnoses, you manifested them so that you can heal them and move into higher states of being.

Sarah Harvey

Chapter 10

Healing Fibromyalgia and Rheumatoid Arthritis Through Food

Over the course of about four years, my health was deteriorating. I had so much pain in my hands and wrists and I was suffering from severe depression. I had brain fog, chronic fatigue and constant headaches that made me feel sick. My legs and arms would be in so much pain all day and night and I would suffer spasms and twitching. I had insomnia - as tired as I was, I just could not sleep!

I was going to the doctor regularly so that he could keep an eye on my worsening conditions. He prescribed me strong anti-depressants and pain killers and sent me for scans and x-rays. Eventually, I was told that I had bad rheumatoid arthritis in both hands, which could be seen on my x-rays and that I had Fibromyalgia. I was given more medication.

Over time, I was like a walking zombie. None of the medication did anything for the pain or my other symptoms. My doctor told me that I would more than likely end up using a stick to walk or be in a wheelchair. That was it.

At this point, I was feeling so depressed that I seriously considered suicide, even though I had four daughters and a thriving business. I just couldn't take any more. I spent my days in pain and crying, not wanting to see anyone, not interested in my children. I was useless to them.

One day though, as I was scrolling through Facebook looking for inspiration, I saw somebody recommend a book by Anthony William, called Medical Medium. I asked one of my daughters for it for Christmas.

Because I was so busy feeling sorry for myself while looking after my children and running a restaurant and Bed and Breakfast in France seven days a week, it actually took me a year to get around to picking up the book and reading it.

My goodness, once I picked it up and started reading it, I couldn't put it down. It explained so much. Other people had gone through the same as me and had completely healed themselves, just by changing their diet!

Over the next three months, I started to do a complete detox. I had already been a vegetarian for twenty-five years; I was now going to become vegan. I spent twenty-eight days eating only fresh fruit and vegetables, having smoothies and taking a few supplements. I was eating as high vibrational food as possible and organic as much as I could afford.

The change in my health in those first four weeks was incredible. I managed to come off all my medication and my depression disappeared. I was able to think more clearly, had more energy and I was getting good night's sleep, every night. It was amazing! After three months, I had healed my body of all signs of Fibromyalgia and had no pain whatsoever.

This was four years ago and I haven't looked back. I started a new life in the UK with my children and have a new job. I can out-walk my kids and I have a future to look forward to that doesn't involve wheelchairs and sticks.

Pharmaceutical medication is not the future. We need to take back control of our body and our health and reduce the toxic load place upon it from today's modern life. I don't take my health for granted any more. I never buy cleaning products with chemicals in, soaps, shampoos, washing powders and all my products are all organic and natural. I buy organic produce as much as possible and I regularly undertake a full detox, involving eating only fruit and vegetables, no processed food. I can honestly say I have never felt better.

Meat comes from animals that have led a frightened, painful, uncared-for life. When they are sent to slaughter and experience terror, the cells in their bodies change. They become low vibrational food and we are ingesting that. Dairy; milk and cheese, as well as eggs, are all virus feeding products. Eggs feed cancer cells and tumours. Milk is produced by cows to feed calves and produce hefty young cows in a small amount of time. Why do we need to be consuming that?

We have all been subjected to so many chemicals all our lives, from vaccinations, to chemicals in processed foods, sprays on crops, mercury in amalgams and the pollution that is falling from the sky above us. We need to take back control and treat our bodies with as much respect as possible. I never thought I would still be here after suffering so much pain and depression, but here I am, loving life, feeling great, and watching three grandchildren growing up.

Teresa Harris

Chapter 11

Healing Fibromyalgia
Naturally

My knowledge of natural health started way back in my late teens (I'm fifty-five now!). I loved natural health shops and their delicious goodies that I could snack on; vegetarian options in the chiller and Rye bread which I felt better eating, instead of the over-processed white flour and additives in white packaged loaves. I also loved using essential oils and skin products without toxins, or so I thought.

After a very challenging sixteen years; divorce, bankruptcy, loss, caught up in the benefits system, moving home seven times and a serious lack of money, oh yes, and three children, I was diagnosed with Fibromyalgia, stress and anxiety. Probably not a total surprise as I had been in considerable body pain and had endless sleepless nights for about ten of those sixteen years!

Having finally had a diagnosis for the pain, and being offered a variety of prescription drugs, I left the Rheumatologists office, with prescription notes in hand, sat in my car and cried! Was this how it is going to be now, a lifetime of tablets just to function in 'normal' life? I didn't want to take pharmaceutical drugs all my life and needed to know what I could do for myself. Where to start, it's a minefield of information out there? It can all get very overwhelming. But, start I did, determined to find options that wouldn't involve popping pills, masking the REAL cause

Firstly, I knew that nothing I had was dangerous, only frustrating, as the aches and pains affected pretty much every moment of every day, and a good night's sleep was a very rare occurrence. It was hard to get going in the morning with the stiffness and the brain fog. It would have been so easy just to stay in bed, if it weren't for my beautiful children and the fact that I had made a decision quite some time ago, that no matter how bad I felt each day, I would still get up and get on with my day, no matter what.

I made the decision that I really needed to do something to ease the pain as I still refused to take tablets, so I decided it was time to get walking. I always loved walking, but it's so hard to 'force' yourself to do exercise, or anything for that matter, when you feel rubbish, literally. However, I knew that if I didn't, nothing was going to change.

Every night as I went to bed, I would lay out my walking gear over a chair ready for the morning. As I was usually awake early anyway, I decided to get up and out before the kids got up. I would walk for about an hour, blasting great uplifting, happy tunes in my ears as I went. It took about ten days of doing this before I felt the real benefit. I had less pain during the day and I was sleeping a little better, as the aching in my bones and muscles was less too. It was a great response for just simply walking. So that got me thinking, what else could I do? This is when things got even more interesting.

I love research, and we have the world at our fingertips, so I spent a great deal of time, months, years, in fact, researching Fibromyalgia, sleep issues, natural pain relief, the list goes on and on. I even became a Certified Life Coach, mainly so I could coach myself back to health. This was really useful, as it helped me with goal setting and planning, as well as keeping me on track and very focused on my natural health and wellbeing journey, which is really important for healing.

I studied Reiki, becoming a Reiki Master, and then became a Reconnective Healing Practitioner so that I could understand how energy works and then use it on myself. What an amazing tool. A simple technique that worked really well for me, and continues to do so, is to rub my hands briskly together for about thirty seconds, then place my now 'buzzing' hands over an area of unease or pain. This felt very comforting and is a natural instinct as a child with pain, earache or tummy ache.

Then Transcendental Meditation found me via a really good friend who was an Advanced Clinical Hypnotherapist. We went together and did an intensive weekend course, which totally turned me around. I now have a wonderful tool to ground and centre me twice a day, so that I don't get overly stressed.

By this time, I was beginning to fall in love with Me, the real Me, nurturing myself and caring about how I felt, spending time just 'being' without the continual thoughts coming through like a train, what a relief. I sat somewhere quiet and warm, closed my eyes and started taking very slow deep breaths, whilst noticing any tension that was in my body, working down from my head to my toes. I then started to relax that area. This was done within a few minutes and my body learnt to relax and be calm, which was important because of my feeling stressed, anxious or in fear.

This technique can also be done using a pure therapeutic grade essential oil, to anchor the feeling of calm with the aroma of the essential oil. This maximised the process because the smell of the oil rekindles a sense of calm and the brain remembers. Perfect for anxiety attacks or panic attacks.

The next part of this journey was a complete game changer for me. I love essential oils, have done since I was a teenager, so it's no surprise then that I still use them now. But what I found out totally changed my life, my aches and pains, my sleep, and well, just about everything. Like most people, I bought essential oils from the high street, I thought that all oils were the same, how wrong I was. And here's where the research got really interesting. I discovered toxins in the essential oils, skin creams and make-up that I had been using on my skin, as well as in the cleaning and washing products I used around my home and cleaned clothes with. Everything I used contained toxic ingredients.

That was it, what was I doing to my Liver, the hardest working organ in my body? It was working so hard to remove all those toxins from my blood because of the products I was using, it must be exhausted. The more I researched, the more I discovered how to have a toxin-free lifestyle. I now use the safest essential oils to stop any pain in its tracks, I take one of the most natural safest and most effective supplements, use toxin-free and Vegan skincare products, and I now make my own cleaning products around the house.

Today I am pain-free, sleep like a baby, am a Natural Health and Wellbeing Coach and a Clinical Aromatherapist, helping others to learn the benefits of a natural, toxin-free lifestyle.

On a side note, I am now in the middle of the glamorous world of Menopause!! I now have very few, if any, hot flushes or night sweats by nourishing my body with mainly fruit, vegetables, legumes, nuts and seeds. I also fast once a week along with Time Restricted Eating, and I have taken as many toxins out of my life as I can. My liver thanked me, and your liver will thank you!

Kathy Newman

Chapter 12

Healing Fibromyalgia Through Chinese Medicine

I am Consuelo. I am fifty-six years old and live in Barbarroja, Spain.

When I was on my way back home from the supermarket, at the age of twenty-six, I started to feel very tired. So tired in fact, that I just had to sit down in the middle of the street and at the same moment, my young daughter asked me if I could carry her in my arms. I was beyond exhausted.

I felt extreme weakness, which was not normal for me because I did so much. My life had suddenly and abruptly changed. All my muscles ached and I started suffering from fluid retention, insomnia, difficulties with digestion, excessive sensitivities, difficulty thinking in stressful situations and the muscle pains were constant, twenty-four hours a day. I went to the Doctor and he diagnosed me with fibromyalgia.

This diagnosis caused me an inability to take effective action, throughout my life, plus the people around me didn't understand the diagnosis. It was a complicated situation for all.

I had a really sensitive stomach and the anti-inflammatory medications I was given to try and help the fibromyalgia, ended up giving me a stomach ulcer, which perforated.

Every day, I felt so exhausted that I did not know how I was going to get up and this created great insecurity in me, to look for work. I was afraid to go to visit places or meet friends because I could suddenly feel very bad.

For example, one day, in a rehabilitation session for this disease, I was in a hydromassage bathtub. I developed stiffness throughout my body, from the bubbles. Can you imagine that?...

In the end, I stopped doing many things and this created a lot of sadness. The doctors prescribed me antidepressants, but I didn't feel any improvement from them.

It was a long road in search of answers and help. I went to the pain centre in San Vicente but they had no empathy for the patient's suffering, not understanding the extreme emotional and physical sense of fibromyalgia. All medical help failed to relieve my suffering.

After a long time spent looking for help, I turned towards Traditional Chinese Medicine, naturopathy, homeopathy and macrobiotic nutrition. It was very interesting.

The truth is that I have learned a lot from this journey. Above all, changing my diet made me understand the sensitivities I had developed from the digestion of some foods. I cut out lactose and stopped eating processed foods as these caused me bloating, diarrhoea and constipation.

Chinese medicine made me understand that there is a different way of approaching life. Psycho-emotionally I realized that I carried emotions that were not mine. I felt sad all the time but I had nothing going on in my life that would cause me to feel this way. Using Reiki and asking my body if this was my emotion or someone else's, I learnt to separate my emotions and those of others'.

To this day, at fifty-six years old, I still want to learn more. I now know that in this life, your body hurting is not a punishment but quite the opposite. When you listen to your body and accept yourself as you are, the judgments of others become a simple opinion, their opinion. Once we understand this, we can start to feel what our own being is like, without their opinions.

To finish, I will give you some things that I learnt to help the healing process:

- Stop seeking approval from others
- Respect yourself as you are by being the best version of you, in everything you do
- Don't criticize yourself or accept other's criticism of you
- Everything happens for our personal advancement

Consuelo Robles

(Translated from Spanish)

Chapter 13

I'm Not Crazy

S everal years ago, I finally found a gynaecologist who believed I was having some very serious feminine issues even though the endometrial biopsy he performed came back normal. I was twenty-six and had spent the previous three years trying to convince my doctors, who had to answer to insurance companies, to explain how an otherwise healthy young girl whose husband might want more children in the future could possibly be having female problems.

It didn't seem to matter that my previous two pregnancies were complicated and ended in caesareans, with the removal of bits and pieces of my fallopian tubes and ovaries. It also didn't seem to matter that I was allergic to the prescription drug Codeine but still opted to take regular daily doses of Tylenol-3 washed down with shots of alcohol just to take enough of the edge off the pain so I might be able to function for another few hours.

So instead of giving me yet another referral to yet another mental health professional, this surgeon offered to give me a radical hysterectomy without the usual preauthorization required by my insurance company. We agreed that if, after the surgery, the pathology came back clean we would then discuss an appropriate payment plan to cover the cost of the surgery. But he felt strongly that wouldn't be the case. He listened to me and to his gut and he discovered he was correct in doing so.

It turned out that what he pulled out of my abdominal cavity could not be described as any kind of healthy pink human organ, but a black rock hard tumor filled fibrous mass about the size of his fist. I can only describe the pain and discomfort of recovery as a mere twinge compared to the level of daily pain I had experienced for months leading up to the surgery.

I'm not crazy and I can't go through this crap again, was my first thought as I pulled my vehicle into the Northeast parking lot of the college. I was attending nursing school. The program offered a two year Degree in Nursing certificate with an option to transfer into the Bachelors of Nursing program upon completion. It was a very competitive program and only a handful of available slots. Each year hundreds of individuals from the tristate area applied with the knowledge that they would likely have to apply at least two or three times before making the cut. I was one of the few lucky ones who got accepted on my first attempt and the last thing I wanted to do was to lose my position or 3.8 GPA to yet another debilitating mystery illness.

As I struggled through the joint pain and visible tremors triggered by my attempt to gather up my books and head for the lecture hall, I realized with no small amount of discouragement and disbelief, I might really be facing some serious health challenges again. But unlike the symptoms of the endometriosis, I had experienced a couple of years before, these new symptoms seemed vague and hard to pin down to any one thing. For example, I couldn't seem to get more than a couple of hours of sleep a night. And that seemed impossible because after a day of college classes, home-schooling the kids and tending bar on the swing shift, I should have slept like a baby. I was also experiencing severe joint pain, headaches, anxiety, and a kind of nervous shakiness that left my heartbeat elevated and my body week and soaked in perspiration.

I really feared that if I went to the doctors, I would definitely be labelled as a hypochondriac or that they would start me on a regiment of pharmaceuticals. I didn't want either to happen for a variety of reason, but I had to do something or I wasn't going to be able to finish the last six months of the nursing program.

I made an appointment with the campus nurse practitioner. I didn't know what to expect but what I found was a caring and compassionate woman who was really ahead of her time. She listened to my complaints, took note of my life's circumstances, ran the usual tests to rule out the usual maladies, and then gave me a diagnosis. She explained to me that she believed I had fibromyalgia and we could approach it in one of two ways. With the first way, I could start a regiment of SSRI antidepressants, prescription pain medications, and psychological therapy (in the mid '90s fibromyalgia was believed to be a kind of delusional mental disorder by many and not the autoimmune disease we know it to be today). As for the second option, which she believed was a more appropriate course to take with regards to any autoimmune issue, she explained I would need to make some serious lifestyle changes.

I chose option two...of course. Even though option two wasn't the easy button I imagined it to be, it was the healthy long-term solution to a potentially devastating lifelong chronic condition. We started by normalizing my sleep patterns. I was given prescription-grade melatonin for a few weeks while I set about the task of changing my sleeping behaviors. I then had to address my current level of stress as well as my potential future stressors.

I began a meditation practice which led to the important realization that I hated working in a hospital setting where I felt more like a legal drug pusher and less like a potential healer. I also realized that if I continued in this direction, I would be completely burned out within five years and useless to myself and others. In response to this realization, I finished up my nursing program and shifted gears.

I became a tattoo artist and made a happy and successful twenty-year run of it before shifting careers again, transitioning into my current career as a Shamanic practitioner and intuitive advisor. Finally, I had to change my diet. I would need to experiment to see what foods worked for me, otherwise avoiding grains and sugar was a must. Within weeks, I was beginning to feel clear minded, pain-free and energetic again.

It's been well over twenty-five years since that day in the parking lot. I have had a few debilitating flare-ups that have lasted from days to weeks. However, these not so wonderful reminders are usually the result of my own occasional disregard for my dietary requirements or my neglecting the proper management of my stress. When this happens, I re-evaluate my lifestyle choices and make the necessary changes again. But I don't let this discourage me because at the age of fifty when many of my family and friends are taking an average of three to six different types of prescribed pharmaceuticals, I only take the occasional over-the-counter or herbal remedy.

I have a good quality of life and feel great most days. I have been blessed with a never give up attitude and rewarded with help and guidance from people who believed and helped me.

Sigrun R Hornberger

Chapter 14

Thyroid Healing Over Surgery

I was diagnosed with Graves' Disease when I was thirty-one, a year after my dad passed of pancreatic cancer. Now knowing the symptoms, I believe I had Graves' disease or at least an overactive thyroid for many years.

My symptoms weren't always at one given time but scattered over the years which consisted of intolerance to heat and without fail, fainting in the summer months or on holiday. Fatigued and exhaustion, bloating, tummy aches, trapped wind, itchy skin, loose stools, mood swings, dry eye, hair loss, hand tremors, double vision and heart palpitations.

I was put on carbimazole, for my thyroid and beta-blockers for the palpitations. The beta-blockers made me feel worse. I became anxious and groggy.

Being very stubborn, I took myself off the beta-blockers much to my doctors' disapproval and under his supervision, I weaned myself from 40mg of carbimazole down to 10mg, then decided to take myself off them completely. What was the worst that could happen? With the changes I had made, I would either feel better or worse. Luckily, I felt better and I believed the change I had made were making a big and positive impact on my overall health.

I had only been on beta-blockers for a matter of weeks and carbimazole around eighteen months. My doctor/endocrinologist informed me that they only allow medication for a year to eighteen months and then I had to decide if I wanted my thyroid removed or radioactive iodine therapy (RAI), then medication for life.

I've learnt for myself that this isn't a cure for Graves at all, the thyroid is the victim! By going down this road of surgery and radioactive therapy, I could of potentially open myself up to another autoimmune disease, diabetes or even worse, cancer in years to come.

I started to research and it became very clear I had two choices. Stay as I am which was a junk food junkie, binge drinker, overworked business owner; a sad and sick individual, or change my lifestyle for the better. If I just removed as many toxins from my mind, body and skin, I could give my body a chance of doing what it was designed to do. Heal and work optimally.

I changed my diet to whole foods, removed refined sugar, gluten, dairy, soy, processed foods, pork, coffee and alcohol. Smoothies, juices, healthy meals all made from scratch became my new routine. I had dietary advice under a holistic health practitioner and medical nutritionist and used supplements.

I changed my personal care products to Arbonne's who I'm now an ambassador for. I chose this brand because they independently ban over two thousand harmful ingredients and focus on clean beauty backed with scientific results. They personally ticked so many boxes for me.

I use essential oils now too because they help me switch off my mind, help me relax and are cleaner and a toxin-free option to perfumes, car air fresheners, scented candles, cleaning products and plug-in air fresheners.

I started to read personal development books daily, which is part of Arbonne. It's changed my world, my health, my business, my relationships with people, my social life. Taught me to self-care, that I am in control of change in my life in every area, to be present and grateful for absolutely everything.

I am so grateful for having Graves' disease because if someone like me can change, so can you. I've been medication-free for two years, symptom-free and still have my thyroid. I've gone on to study nutrition and work alongside a medical nutritionist within Arbonne to help people learn healthier habits.

Arbonne make no guarantees, results are different for everyone

Thank you to my sister Anne-Marie, it's been great to grow and improve on our health journey together.

Thank you to my cousin Gemma, who informed and educated me that there is another way.

Thank you to Debbie, my homeopath, who guided me to heal me heal.

Thank you to Tara, Medical Nutritionist, for all your help and for helping me to help others.

Thank you to Philip, the top independent health researcher in the UK for all your seminars, chats and knowledge.

Thank you to Kate, Robert and Susan for all that you do to share your knowledge and to help people.

Thank you to everyone who has been part of my healing and journey and supports what I do.

Love and light to you all.

Julie Rose

Chapter 15

A Life of Pain, Brain Fog and Fatigue from Lupus, Turned Around Through Nutrition

I hadn't felt right for at least ten years.

It had started around the time I gave birth to my daughter in 2009. I had Carpal Tunnel Syndrome, chronic shoulder pain, bouts of depression during the pregnancy and post-partum and worsening uncomfortable varicose veins in my legs.

I felt worse again after the birth of my son, four years later. I constantly felt fatigued, enveloped in brain fog and started to experience aches and pains in my body.

Attributing all this to having two young children, especially being an 'older mum' because I had kids at thirty-five and thirty-nine years old, I didn't give it much thought and just accepted that it was part of the parenting process.

Over the years, I developed more on and off pains in the jaw, wrists and knees. Things worsened after June 2015 when my mother died rather suddenly after a botched-up surgery. The grief for the loss of my mother exacerbated the symptoms and it felt like my body was imploding. The brain fog worsened, my memory was terrible and I couldn't remember why I walked into a room, or why I went to the fridge. I was constantly misplacing my car keys and losing parking tickets. I could not do simple math like calculating the change for my purchases.

I was chronically fatigued and looking back, I am sure I dozed off while driving a couple of times. It was scary.

My scalp hurt. Over time my hair thinned and I experienced quite a lot of hair loss. By the time I was diagnosed with Lupus, my hair was thin and brittle (lupus hair) so I just had to cut it short.

The bones!! I never knew bones could ache. I placed a cushion on the driver's seat of my car because my bum bones hurt to sit. It hurt to walk because my feet bones felt like they were grinding into the ground, so I had to walk slowly and gingerly.

My fingers stiffened and swelled one night after a spa treatment and I remember frantically rubbing my fingers with soap to try and remove my wedding ring.

I had a low-grade fever for about two months before having the sense to see a rheumatologist. I told him that I thought I had rheumatoid arthritis; it was September 2016. My rheumatologist ran some tests and informed me that I have Systemic Lupus Erythematosus (SLE) and that my test results were 'off-the-charts' with a dsDNA titre of greater than one thousand international units per milliliter (IU/ml); less than thirty is a negative result and more than seventy is a positive result.

Not long after, I had trouble breathing and was diagnosed with pleural effusion in my left lung, which was complicated with a bout of left basal pneumonia in October 2016. I was prescribed Prednisolone, Mycophenolate Mofetil, antibiotics and Hydroxychloroquine.

I also developed costochondritis. I had stabbing pains in my rib cage which felt like someone was stabbing me with a knife from the inside. I was in so much pain it was unbelievable. Needless to say, it felt like I had hit rock bottom and decided that I'd had enough. I needed to get my life back.

A friend of mine, a health coach, told me about the possibility of healing chronic diseases with food. I dove into research on autoimmunity and functional medicine, and the importance of the right nutrition that our bodies need to thrive. All the functional medicine practitioners I came across described nutrients that the body needs to thrive. I heard the words 'leaky gut' for the first time and learned about the need to heal the gut. I learned there was a range of diets that could heal diseases, whether it was an autoimmune protocol (AIP), ketogenic, paleo or vegan diets.

After reading up on all these diets, one stood out by Doctor Terry Wahls in her book The Wahls Protocol – A Radical New Way to Treat All Chronic Autoimmune Diseases Using Paleo Principles. Doctor Wahls had struggled with a far worse condition than mine because she had Multiple Sclerosis which had deteriorated to the extent that she needed a tilt/recline wheelchair. She experimented with foods on herself over a period of time and healed herself.

I was inspired and decided to do the same. I did my best to follow her diet exactly, fitting in the nine cups a day of vegetables, (Three each of leafy greens, different colours and sulfur-rich vegetables). It was much easier to drink all those greens in smoothies than eat so much food, so I blended and drank my vegetables and fruits.

Later on, I found out about Dr Brooke Goldner who has completely healed herself of Stage four lupus on a vegan diet. She prescribes huge amounts of smoothies, nearly two litres a day (up to 64 ounces a day), and recommends that animal products, added oils and processed foods be removed from the diet. I removed gluten and dairy from my diet and ate wild caught-fish and free-range meat. I even tried to find out what the animals were fed.

This was harder for me as I cook for my family, and it wasn't going to be easy to turn them into vegans. I predominantly eat mostly vegetables with little meat, and decided to increase the volume of smoothies.

Thankfully, I was able to stop the Prednisolone after one year, and then stop the Mycophenolate Metofil a year and a half later because of my health improvements from changing my lifestyle. I now only take one Hydroxychloroquine tablet a day for prognostic purposes.

I moved to the UK and saw a rheumatologist in November 2020. My dsDNA is now down to a "borderline case" at forty-three international units per milliliter (IU/ml). I am also pain and symptom-free, energetic, and feel strong again.

I have been drinking daily green smoothies for almost four and a half years, and firmly believe they have strongly contributed to my healing.

It's not magic, it's about nutrition. In our fast-paced lives, we have forgotten how to eat properly, to consume the nutrients that our bodies need to thrive. Healing takes dedication and time, and a strong desire to heal. I'm still learning and still experimenting.

Fania Koh

Chapter 16

Holistic Nutrition and Therapies Reversed Lupus

I was diagnosed with Lupus in the fall of 1993. A year before my diagnosis, I started experiencing joint pain in my hands and feet. I just thought I may be developing arthritis because genetically from my mom's side of the family, arthritis was very prevalent. I went to see a few doctors, but they found no arthritis.

Later that year, during the summer, I was still experiencing joint pain but now I noticed hair loss, sensitivity to the sun, loss of appetite and flu-like symptoms; extremely high fevers and chills. I went from a size four to a size double zero and weighed ninety pounds. I had no idea what was going on. I felt tired and exhausted all the time. One morning I woke up and when my feet touched the floor, I felt intense pain and weakness. I fell to the floor. It felt like my life-force was sucked out of me. I could barely get myself off the floor and onto my bed. My whole body was in pain, my joints had a lot of inflammation and it felt as if they were being scraped and stabbed by a knife. I was scared. I did not know what was going on with me.

I went to see a doctor. He had no clue what was going on with me either. He said it could be the flu. I was not satisfied with that answer. I knew there was something else was going on. For the past year, I felt my body changing. I kept experiencing pain, so the diagnosis of the flu made no sense to me. One doctor recommended I go see a psychiatrist. Since the doctors I went to see had no clue. I started researching different medical journals, articles, and books about different illnesses with similar symptoms. I finally came across an autoimmune disease called Systemic Lupus Erythematosus (SLE). After learning about SLE, there was no doubt in my mind that I had Lupus. The next day I called my dermatologist to schedule an appointment. During my research, I had read that both a dermatologist and a rheumatologist can perform the test for SLE. My results came back positive for SLE.

I contacted the Lupus Foundation of America to get a list of rheumatologists who treat the illness and get more information about the disease. They were fantastic, sent me lots of information and told me about their local support group. I found a wonderful rheumatologist in my area from the list of doctors' the Lupus Foundation shared with me. In my first week of being diagnosed, I started learning and reading all I could find about the disease. I went to some of the Lupus foundation's local support groups in NYC and met others who had similar issues to mine. I got a wealth of information from that support group; they were extremely helpful.

A week after my diagnosis, I had my first bad lupus flare-up. I felt like I was dying, the pain all over my body was unbearable; I was so weak! I couldn't stand up, I had a high fever, and couldn't keep any food down.

I could not walk to the bathroom because I felt so weak, so I would crawl on the floor, throw up in the bathroom, and then lay on the bathroom floor until my dad came home. My dad would pick me up off the floor and drive me to the doctor. He had to carry me into the doctor's office because I was too weak to walk. I was admitted immediately to the hospital because I was having a bad flare-up. Lupus was beating me up and I was scared that this was the way my life was going to be from now on. I have never felt so helpless in my entire life! I was discharged after several days' stay in the hospital.

Still, I kept getting sick and having many flare-ups. My doctor put me on high levels of prednisone and wanted to put me on other stronger medication. I refused the other medications and fought with him to take me off prednisone. He slowly reduced my dose, until I was completely off it.

I was constantly in and out of the hospital, sometimes staying a week, only to return the following week. Lupus attacked my heart twice, causing me to have surgery and four stents inserted. Lupus can cause several heart conditions and it left me with a condition called atherosclerosis, a type of Coronary Artery Disease. Atherosclerosis is a disease in which plaque builds up inside your arteries. Atherosclerosis can lead to serious problems, including heart attack, stroke, or even death.

I was desperate. I started researching alternative therapies and diets for Lupus. During this time, I decided to go back to school to study holistic nutrition and other holistic therapies. (Holistic nutrition, Herbalism, Traditional Chinese Medicine [TCM], Ayurveda, exercise, Usui Reiki, and eventually became a Reiki master. Chakra Healing, meditation, and flower essences, as well as mindset techniques, and stress reduction exercise, and working on my emotional traumas.)

I started to change my diet and take yoga classes. I switched to an anti-inflammatory diet, I stopped eating foods with gluten, cut out dairy, eggs, and processed foods. I started juicing and eating more fruits and vegetables, I got rid of sugar, ate lean protein, drank a lot of water, slept at least seven to eight hours, tapped into my spirituality, and incorporated herbal therapies and exercise as well. I also had to repair my gut because my gut health was horrible. I began healing my deep-rooted traumas and started my healing journey. I started to feel better and was able to do things I could not do before.

Two years after making all the changes, my rheumatologist did another test for Lupus and was no longer able to find it in my system. Seventeen years later I am still Lupus free and now I am a health coach, nutritionist, and healer who helps others with Lupus to reverse it, just like I did. Now I can kickbox, climb and hike and do things I thought I would never be able to do again. All the hard work and time I invested in my health was worth it.

Yvette Laboy

Lupus Wellness Coach

Chapter 17

Life-Changing ME

I was diagnosed with Myalgic Encephalomyelitis/Chronic Fatigue Syndrome (ME/CFS) and Generalised Anxiety in Autumn 2016, aged forty, after collapsing at the end of a triathlon, my first – ironically, I'd been trying to improve my health!

I'd spent the week before the triathlon in high anxiety, which had been creeping up over the previous few years. My step-dad had had a heart attack and I was also terrified about the upcoming triathlon. It turned out to be the straw that broke the camel's back. After years of pushing through almost constant tiredness and frequent illness that first started with Glandular Fever at age seventeen, which I struggled to recover from, I was diagnosed with Post Viral Fatigue. I just never seemed right from then on.

The CFS diagnosis itself was traumatic, involving numerous doctor and hospital visits, with many tests. I was so exhausted that I could barely function. I was having heart palpitations, regular panic attacks, extreme anxiety, exhaustion, headaches, feeling faint, being unable to walk and so many more symptoms. The diagnosis was both a relief and devastating, as I was told all I could do was learn to manage it. But I rejected that prognosis from the start. I wasn't going to just manage it, this was not how my life was going to be. I was going to recover.

I started searching the internet and came across The Optimum Health Clinic, run by people who took a holistic approach to recovery and recovered from CFS. I immediately started working with their Nutrition and Psychology departments. This was my first introduction to healing CFS from a mind/body perspective - which my instinct had always felt was the way forward. I learnt about how important it was for my body to be in a 'healing state' i.e. relaxed in both body and mind. I began meditating and learnt how to use EFT (Emotional Freedom Technique) to help process emotions. Basically, what goes on in our minds directly affects our physiology.

I had also reluctantly started seeing a psychiatrist regarding the anxiety and panic attacks as they were causing me to spiral down into more exhaustion, leading to me being totally bed bound for about three months. Despite never being keen on pharmaceutical drugs, I was desperate for some relief and have to say the antidepressants and anti-anxiety medication made a huge difference, allowing my exhausted body respite from the panic attacks.

I also began removing as many toxins as I could. I started with my diet, removing alcohol, caffeine, refined sugar, processed food, gluten and dairy, then moved onto cleaning and personal products.

Over the next couple of years, I worked with various people to support my healing. Each took a holistic approach and whilst they saw CFS very much as a physical illness, they also believed it to be the body displaying physical symptoms as a result of being in a prolonged state of stress and becoming stuck in what the Optimum Health Clinic describe as the 'maladaptive stress response', basically the autonomic nervous system is 'stuck' in fight / flight / freeze and causing a cascade of symptoms throughout every system in the body.

I learnt that it was my responsibility to heal myself; which was both scary (what if I can't do it?) and empowering (it's down to me so I have control). Also, our bodies' ability to heal is the most natural thing in the world. As long as we're giving it the best conditions for that healing to happen. So, I stopped fighting my body. I stopped fighting CFS and learned to see them as friends, sending me symptoms to let me know that something was wrong. My body wanted the best for me!

I began to slow down, treat myself better, get grateful for the small things in life, be more present and find the positives in life rather than getting caught up in the unhelpful negative thoughts. I needed to listen to my body and the messages it was giving me. To see symptoms as feedback rather than something 'bad'. Basically to accept and surrender to where I was, whilst doing the things I knew would support my body in healing; meditation, mindfulness, resting, pacing my activity, getting out of my crazy brain and living more from my heart, detoxing (things like Epsom salts baths, dry brushing, fermented foods and specific herbal supplements), being present, finding joy and the biggie - realising there was nothing I needed to fix, change or improve about myself, instead to accept myself exactly as I am - the good, the bad and the ugly. Which is a much less stressful and conflicting place to be. Not that I always managed to do all these things. I had many times where I ended up in a total mess!

I slowly improved to be able to walk again (slowly and not too far), drive locally, socialise more and do things like picking my kids up from school, make dinner, do the laundry etc. I was lucky enough to have a LOT of help from my husband, my mum and a nanny who helped out a couple of days as we had young children, aged six and eight when I first became ill. I started working from home for myself part-time, which gave me a positive focus.

But I wasn't fully recovered and needed to pace myself, resting every afternoon and cancelling plans. I would still have crashes now and then. By Autumn 2019, I was sliding backwards again. I was working more, pushing myself again and getting stressed. Our nanny had left to go to New Zealand so I had less help around the house, and my husband was busy starting a new business. Then in March 2020, when I was already struggling, COVID came along and I had my first anxiety attack since those early days (I'd been off my medication for about a year or so). Nothing I did seemed to make a difference, I slid into a downward spiral of severe anxiety, depression and fatigue, again ending up virtually bedbound.

I went back to what had helped me before. I re-focussed on meditation, went back to having coaching to help me see the unhelpful patterns I was still running in my thoughts and underlying beliefs. And yet, I hit rock bottom prior to going to Cornwall for a family holiday after lockdown finished, so I went back to my psychiatrist and back onto medication. Again, that immediately helped calm my nervous system and allowed me to properly rest, regaining a little strength and positivity. Since early July (it's now the end of December 2020) I've slowly been improving again.

I've also recently tested positive for Lyme's Disease and various co-infections so am about to embark on a lengthy herbal protocol to help my body eliminate these.

I've learnt so much from this relapse. The key things have been really learning to live more from my heart. I start every morning with a heart meditation where I invite love, compassion, gratitude and joy into my heart; tell myself mantras like "I love you, I'm here for you" and also thank my body for healing and visualise myself healthy. I now see my thoughts as separate to myself, learning to observe them with curiosity rather than getting caught up and overwhelmed by them. I've also learnt to see the patterns of thoughts and beliefs that I run and how I can replace these with more helpful ones.

So, what would I say are the biggest things that are helping me? Living in a state of acceptance of everything as it is, trusting that my body will heal, accepting and allowing all of my emotions instead of pushing them away and fearing them, purposely cultivating feelings of gratitude, joy and love, and learning to live and love a simpler life, from my heart. And above all to be true to myself and to love and accept myself exactly as I am.

Recently I've started painting and share both my art and some of my musings about healing on my Instagram page. Both of which I also find hugely therapeutic.

Hazel Stinson

Chapter 18

From Pain to Peace

I loved my life. I had a beautiful family, a loving husband, a lovely home in an idyllic town. This was what I had always wanted, planned and created. A career in engineering and teaching engineering at a college was hugely satisfying for me. I was physically active, fit, strong and vibrant. My three children had all left the nest and were making their own way in the world. Retirement was only a few years away and my husband and I were looking forward to the freedom years with eager anticipation.

This beautiful fairytale came crumbling down in 2015, beginning with the sudden passing of my beloved mother. She was my best friend and my champion. The grief of her loss permeated my very core. Along with the sadness came the huge responsibility of being the executor of her estate, dealing with a lifetime's worth of possessions and family tensions that inevitably came to the surface. I tried to manage all this, with my high standard of fairness and attention to detail, over a long distance and while continuing with my work as a college instructor. I was sad, stressed and hardly sleeping.

A year later, just after I turned fifty, I was in the final stages of the very physical and emotional work of divesting my mother's home of its contents and preparing it for market. After long days of packing up, cleaning and painting, I noticed some pain in my shoulder. I thought it was an old rotator cuff injury resurfacing, but the pain was much more intense.

The next day it happened to the other shoulder. I went to physiotherapy but strangely, the pain would move to different joints. One day it would be my left shoulder, another day it was my right elbow, or my wrist. Like a Voodoo doll being stuck with pins, the pain migrated around my body.

A few weeks later my feet started to hurt, so I got fitted for orthotics. Then my knuckles turned a strange purple colour and my fingers began to swell. My knees swelled up as if there were golf balls beneath the skin. With a sudden crack one day, pain set into my jaw.

I knew this had to be related to the physical and emotional stress and lack of sleep.

By this time, I had completed my executor duties and I thought, with the stress behind me and a vacation from work, I would be fine a few weeks.

In fact, I got worse. Three months from the onset of symptoms, I could barely walk. I couldn't make a fist with my hands. My grip was so weak, I could barely squeeze shampoo out of the bottle. Fear crept in as I wondered if I was ever going to get well.

Of course, I was spending a lot of time with Dr Google. The symptoms were sounding suspiciously like rheumatoid arthritis, an autoimmune condition. I really didn't know much about autoimmune disease. It wasn't in my family and I wasn't close to anyone who had been diagnosed with one.

It would be a wait of several months to see a rheumatologist. In the meantime, my family doctor suggested that I could experiment with food. She explained that joint pain was often related to food triggers. I honestly didn't think there could possibly be a link between the food I ate and joint pain, but I was desperate and willing to try anything.

I am forever grateful to my amazing doctor who changed the trajectory of my life. Without her, I may have gone a completely different route. At a time when I felt powerless, she gave me hope that there was something I could do.

With this change in perspective, at a rock-bottom moment, curled up in pain, I MADE A DECISION: I was going to do everything I could to get my life and freedom back again. Disability and pain were NOT how I wanted to spend my life! I was going to figure this out and not stop until I did.

Being an engineer, I put engineering problem solving and project management skills to work and began researching how to heal rheumatoid arthritis as naturally as possible.

Knowing stress had been a big trigger, it made sense to evaluate stress in my life. Also knowing that food had the power to harm and the power to heal, I experimented with what I ate and how I ate. I started by eliminating gluten, dairy and sugar then moved to an autoimmune protocol paleo food plan.

Stories of healing became my inspiration. I changed my lifestyle by prioritizing sleep, getting gentle movement, regular massage and reducing stress. I tracked my food and symptoms making charts and graphs so I could visually see the progress I was making. I began trusting my body and my inner wisdom to guide me in the right direction.

Week by week I began to improve. Knowing that there was something I COULD DO to help alleviate the symptoms, moved me from feeling like a victim to being in charge of my healing. What a feeling of empowerment!

Over the next weeks and months, I continued on my quest for health, trying different lifestyle changes, tracking symptoms, and healing. I discovered functional medicine and got down to healing root causes.

By the time I saw a rheumatologist and was officially diagnosed with rheumatoid arthritis, I was well on my way with healing naturally. I knew masking symptoms with medications was not the route I would take and I didn't want the side effects that went with them. Luckily, my rheumatologist was supportive of my approach, although he could only offer medications if my symptoms got worse.

My symptoms didn't get worse, but while I was significantly better, my healing plateaued.

I began studying the connections between emotions and illness and was fascinated that there were emotional patterns that went along with rheumatoid arthritis. Common emotions associated with rheumatoid arthritis are resentment, feeling like the weight of the world is on your shoulders, and feeling victimized.

Trauma, especially childhood trauma can be associated with many illnesses. The Adverse Childhood Events (ACE) score can show a relationship between childhood events and chronic illness. I learned that trauma doesn't even have to be that severe to have an impact on health.

My childhood wasn't traumatic, but it wasn't perfect either. I developed feelings of unworthiness at a young age, leading to people-pleasing and perfectionism as I got older. I realized how a lifetime of never feeling good enough had impacted my health, physically and emotionally.

Old childhood feelings of unworthiness came to the surface again with the family tensions that arose after my mother's passing. Although I appeared to be successful on so many levels on the outside, these feelings were still in my subconscious mind and stored in my body.

Looking back, I realized that I had been carrying tension in my body my whole life. Achy shoulders, neck pain, and tendonitis had showed up many times over the years. Rheumatoid arthritis was my awakening: my body telling me I had to finally deal with the emotions. I had to learn to love myself from the inside out and reprogram my mind.

Once I really began using mind-body medicine techniques like meditation, journaling, EFT tapping, and energy medicine, and addressing limiting beliefs from childhood, my healing resumed.

Using many different healing modalities starting with mindset and incorporating food, movement, sleep, stress reduction and fostering positive relationships eventually I reversed the symptoms of rheumatoid arthritis.

Now, as long as I listen to my body and provide the right physical, emotional and spiritual environment, I am pain-free and vibrant … with no medications. Most importantly, I became my own champion. The voice in my head is now loving and supportive.

My personal experience with illness and healing led me to leave my thirty year engineering career and become a functional medicine certified health coach. Now I help other women find freedom so that they never need to miss out on life again because of joint pain.

Jane Hogan

Chapter 19

Healing Three Autoimmune Conditions

My healing journey started more than two decades ago, but I didn't start to truly heal until recently. I was first diagnosed with Vitiligo in my late twenties, then Hashimoto's in my late thirties and Addison Disease in my early fifties. Each illness brought many different symptoms.

Vitiligo was probably the most detrimental to my overall health because it affected my emotional state. If you have vitiligo then you know what I am talking about, it's an embarrassing disease. I am white, but have olive colored skin which darkened in the summer months. So, as the sun tanned my skin, the white spots would appear whiter. I dreaded summers and stopped wearing shorts, dresses and short sleeve shirts. I hid from the world during those months. Little by little, more white spots appeared and after my mother passed away, I lost large patches of pigments all over my body. This was a clear indication how stress played a huge role in my health.

The Hashimoto's symptoms included thinning hair, cold extremities, exhaustion, brain fog and muscle and joint pain and I felt sick all the time. Medication did relieve many of my symptoms, but unfortunately, I had to keep increasing my medication every five to ten years.

Addison's Disease is the most serious of all my diagnosis. This is a disorder where the adrenal glands stop producing important hormones the body needs. I was told my body can't handle stress and I could go into crisis if I were to become very sick or have some kind of accident. The year leading up to this diagnosis I was very weak and frail. I lost a lot of weight and literally couldn't walk or stand for very long. I knew something was terribly wrong.

Yet, when I was given this diagnosis, I was not afraid. I didn't become hysterical with a third diagnosis or being told I would be on steroids for the rest of my life. I actually remained very calm and just accepted it. You see, two months before, I read a book by Dr Joe Dispenza called *You are the Placebo*. This book was the true beginning of my healing. Dr Dispenza wrote in his book that if people can be healed by the simple act of their mind believing a pill can heal them, why not just change the way you think without the placebo pill. The main premise of the book is to explain that we can rewire our brains into stopping and reversing illnesses. When we meditate and slow down, our brain waves become more coherent and can send the correct messages to the rest of the body.

I went deep into meditation. The change in me was dramatic. It wasn't just meditating; it was knowing what my emotions were doing to my body. I learned to let go of the strong negative emotions that had become a part of me. I began studying the Law of Attraction and realized that my delay in healing was simple, I was vibrating at a low vibration for years. My sadness and anger towards the illnesses were actually keeping me sick. Once I realized that my thoughts and emotions were sending out these low vibrations, I consciously made a switch to bring myself into a state of higher frequencies. This helped bring my body, mind and spirit into balance.

Meditation also seemed to bring me effortless answers to my healing questions. Even before this time, I never believed that I would be sick for the rest of my life. So, I never stopped looking for answers. Yet, it wasn't until I started meditating and giving thanks every day for what I had in my life, that the right answers started coming to me. I would come out of a mediation and go on the internet and boom, people and knowledge I had never seen before would show up. I didn't realize it at the time, but I was changing my energy field. My own vibrations started attracting the things I needed in my life. I made a decision to quit my stressful job and focus on me.

I learned about energy medicine and it resonated with me so much that I started studying and now, years later, I have become a Reiki master helping others gain balance in their lives. We are all made up of energy and it plays a role in how our bodies heal. Our emotions directly affect our energy systems so it is important to work on emotions in our life, such as fear, anger, worry and sadness. Reiki, along with qigong, acupuncture, and yoga are great healing modalities that help bring the body into a place of peace and harmony.

A major factor for my healing came when I found Anthony Williams, aka the *Medical Medium*. His statement that autoimmune diseases are not our bodies attacking itself, rather it is a virus with toxins that go into our organs, skin, joints, muscles, nervous systems and brain. This was a game changer. No longer did I think my body was faulty, but there were real culprits to blame.

Williams believes the Epstein Barr virus is the cause of many chronic illnesses. I stopped feeding the virus food it loved like eggs, dairy, gluten and corn and replaced them with healing foods. Food became my new medicine and I filled my body with all of God's bounty. I truly believe drinking celery juice (which the *Medical Medium* wrote a whole book on) brought my body back to life. It can actually restore the adrenal glands!

Detoxing was also very important so my liver could work at its best. Supplements such as Zinc, Vitamin C, and B12 are important for immune support. I learned that vitiligo is likely caused by aluminum combined with a virus that oxidizes in the skin. If you do nothing else, read his book *The Medical Medium, Secrets behind Chronic and Mystery Illness.*

Within a few months of combining all my protocols, my energy levels drastically improved, my hair was thick again, the brain fog had lifted and I knew I was on my way to healing. Improvements continue to this day; my thyroid medication has been lowered twice and my numbers continue to improve. I still take medication for the Addison's but I know my adrenals are working better, I can feel it. Most people with Addison's take multiple medications throughout the day. I am only on one now and at the lowest possible dosage. I know that at some point, I will safely be off this medicine, with the support of my doctor.

My real joy came a year after incorporating these protocols into my life. I was outside enjoying my backyard and swimming in my pool. This was something I hadn't done in years because I didn't want anyone to see my skin. Now, I didn't care. I soaked up the beautiful healing sun's rays and relaxed in the water. When I showered later that day I looked down at my skin and saw little brown freckles had popped up in my white spots! I didn't mention earlier that I had spent years trying everything to heal my skin. I tried ointments and creams, steroid shots, UVB light treatments, laser therapy and more. Years of stress and time and money and nothing brought back my skin color. Yet, that day, just sitting and enjoying my life my skin started its return. It's been almost two years since then and my skin continues to improve. Many spots have completely filled in and I am patiently waiting for it all to be perfect again.

My message to anyone out there trying to heal is that your body can heal! It's designed to heal and keep us healthy. We know this already yet have somehow allowed ourselves to believe that it can't happen. Simply explained, if we get a cut the body goes into action and heals up the cut as quickly as it can. The same is true for any illness. The problem is our bodies have become overburdened with toxins, processed foods, stress and pathogens. All the healing modalities I have mentioned here assist the body in its own natural healing. Our own bodies are the best healers in the world. If you would like to find out more information about my healing journey and how it can help you, please visit my website and Instagram page.

Christine Barrett

Cancer

"Healing doesn't mean the damage never existed. It means the damage no longer controls our lives."

Unknown

Chapter 20

"Juicy Life" Healing

Hello friend... the following is wisdom I am sharing with you about my life journey of my mom dying of cancer and ten years later me manifesting a cancer scare in my own body and healing it and now helping thousands of clients self-heal their bodies.

Let me start by saying... If you have some serious illness in your body, then do not allow fear to paralyze you. You can heal all sickness from your body with the power of nutrition, cleansing and your mind belief system. If your body is in DIS–EASE, you likely have too many toxins and your body's own self-healing mechanism can no longer function. You will need to cleanse your body as fast as possible. Disease is created in your energetic body and this sickness energy shows itself somewhere in your physical body as blocked energy / sickness.

To create a deeper natural healing and to get rid of these ailments once and for all, you will need to dive deep into your soul and your heart. You will need to start a deeper cleansing and a vegetable juicing detox program incorporating energetic and mindful healings, meditation, self-love, massages, movement, forgiveness and a holistic raw food nutrition program to infuse the body with a massive amount of nutrition and healing.

Take your health into your hands and heal yourself right now. You have the power in your hands, you just have to remember that you do. I am here to remind you. So, take the baton and claim your health and healing right now! You deserve it. You are worth it. It is your birth right to be healthy and happy and safe on this planet. Claim your birth right and live it. I am here supporting you all the way!

Sixteen years ago my mom was diagnosed with cancer and died within three months. She went from a "healthy vibrant woman" to death extremely quickly. Was it the cancer that got her or was it the diagnosis from her doctor that she had three months left and the ingrained belief that cancer is an instant death sentence?

I feel the latter….

My mom's diagnosis and death launched me into the world of self-healing, detox and juicy raw food. I began to learn everything I could about superhero level food, self-healing the body and never getting sick. Food is our fuel and it can be "our medicine" or "our poison", and we get to choose.

I also started to believe that I was slowly being chased by cancer and it would one day get me like it got my mom. This motivated me to learn everything I could about self-healing the body.

As we believe, we make it so….

About ten years after my mom's death, two different natural health scans showed that I had some blocked energy / inflammation / heat above my right breast and it was possible that it could be the early stages of breast cancer.

Even though I knew that this potential cancer was self-created in my body with the power of my mind and my environment… Even though I knew my body had an innate self-healing system inside that is working on my healing twenty-four-seven… Even though I knew that I am the creator of my reality and that I choose to sit in the driver's seat of my life… And even though I knew that the ability to self-heal myself is completely up to me and up to my thoughts…. I was still scared.

I decided to put into practice everything I knew about self-healing, creating my new reality and shifting my belief systems. I chose to self-heal myself through cleansing and detoxing my body first because I knew it is the only way to truly heal anything.

I grew my own wheatgrass and juiced it daily. I grew sunflower sprouts and other sprouts for juices, smoothies and salads. I ate as clean and green as possible. I focused on alkalizing my body with alkaline water, alkaline veggie juices, fresh vegetables and no chemical food. I did a liver and kidney detox flush where I drank apple juice, took phos liquid and activated magnesium to flush stones out of my organs. I did a metal detox cleanse. I did colonics and enemas. I went to saunas, infrared saunas and had detox cleansing baths to get the toxins out through my skin and sweat.

I sat in sister circles to cry, release emotions and feel loved / supported. I boosted up my vitamin and food nutrition content so I could replenish my body. I drank lots and lots of liquids to flush out my system. I ate mainly freshly picked raw vegetables. I listened to empowering audiobooks to help me shift my mindset into more positivity and confidence in my self-healing journey.

Six months later... I had a biopsy and it was negative, of course. I know now that I went through this crazy journey so I could help others know their worth, their inner power and their ability to have a healthy thriving extraordinary life. All we have to do is BELIEVE!!! Really, really believe in ourselves and in our ability to believe things we wish into being.

Read this to yourself now:

I believe in me. I believe in me. I believe in me. I trust in me. I trust in my ability to create my self-healing. I trust in my ability to create a beautiful life for me. I trust in me. I trust in the I AM consciousness that is me. I am creator. I am it. There is nothing else. There is no one else. I am. Only. I am. I am fully in charge of how I express my I AM creator energy. I am sick or I am healthy. I am happy or I am miserable. I am empowered or I am a victim. I am in charge. I let go of the programming and conditioning put on me. I let go of my own limiting beliefs. I let go of lack and it's not possible. I create my life as if my life is depending on it. Because it is... I believe in me. I believe in me. I believe in me.

I send you so much love and faith... and I believe you can do anything.

Sadly, my mom died with most of her song still inside her and so this is why I am sharing my story with you today. I want every one of you to sing your song and live your fully self-expressed life on this planet.

Heal yourself, empower yourself and live your most fully self-expressed extraordinary life now.

I love you...

Petra "EatJuicy"

Juicy Living School

Raw Vegan Chef, Cleanse & Detox Expert,

Writer & Inspirational Speaker

Author of

- *"KISS ME LIKE THIS - Men's Manual to What Women Really Want and Finding Your Inner Confidence"*
- *"I AM AMAZING - A No Nonsense Self Love Guide to Remember Your Greatness and Rock Out Your Life"*
- CZECH TRANSLATION: *"JA JSEM UZASNA - Zaruceny Navod Na Sebelasku, Ktery Ti Pripomene Tvoji Dokonalost A Zmeni Tvuj Zivot"*
- *"DETOX ME JUICY - The 7 Day Juicy Food Cleanse to Lose Weight, Youthen & Heal Your Body of Everything"*
- *"5 THINGS I LOVE ABOUT YOU - A Guide for You to Heal Your Relationships with Everyone"*

Chapter 21

Cancer? Me? Noooo!

I see two tumors on your left breast. She said, "one in situ and one an invasive ductal carcinoma." She said it bluntly. No feelings. No compassion. Nothing. Just straight to the facts. "We are going to have to do a biopsy to see if it is cancer or not, but to me, it looks like it's malignant." She said it in a rush, like she was in a hurry to be somewhere else. That is how I found out that I had breast cancer. October 1, 2015. I'll never forget the date.

I was seized by an emotion that was rather unusual for me, one that I had never experienced before. It was not fear, as such. I have no words that can really describe it. Besides, I was incredibly surprised by the news because I had been teaching about the power of the mind for thirty years. I started learning about it early in my life, at the age of nineteen, when I was diagnosed with a different terminal condition. I healed myself then...I did not die as I was supposed to, as the medical profession, including my parents who were both physicians, thought I would. That so-called illness brought me a fascinating lesson in life, that we can heal ourselves by using our mind. So, I wasn't afraid. I knew I could heal myself. But nonetheless, I had questions. Many questions.

How could I have cancer if I was the one teaching others how to heal themselves?

How could I have cancer if I knew what the real cause was?

How could I have cancer if I was eating organic food, even before it was common?

How could I have breast cancer if I had breastfed my two boys for years, not months?

How could I have cancer if I was in a loving, respectful thirty-year relationship with the father of my kids?

That day I was at the Cleveland Clinic just doing a general checkup, one that just happened to include a routine mammogram. I had no symptoms whatsoever. The doctor congratulated me on my good health after all the test results were back. "Mrs Stone you are healthier than I am," he said, "congratulations!" I even posted that on Facebook. I was so proud of myself! I was fifty-eight years old and in excellent health. And then, a couple of weeks later came the cancer diagnosis.

I was born in Mexico City in 1956. My parents were gynecologists. They had a small clinic where they mostly delivered babies, which meant I grew up believing strongly in conventional medicine. But my first fatal diagnosis, a "progressive posterior cerebral arteritis" that resulted in a temporary loss of eyesight, led to me being prescribed exceedingly high doses of cortisone.

Six months later, that cortisone destroyed the head of my right femur. I then spent two long years in bed before I was able to get a hip replacement. That is when I lost faith in modern medicine and everything else. The high dosage was considered medically justified due to the original diagnosis. How could they have gotten it so wrong? Even after I regained my eyesight, the damage to my femur was permanent and after three difficult surgeries, I ended up without a hip replacement and with my right leg six inches shorter than my left. That's how I still am today.

When you learn about the power of your mind, you understand that we are responsible for everything that happens to us. We are not victims of an external circumstance or power. We cause our experiences, both the good and the so-called bad. Once I understood this and many other things about the mind, I led a "normal" life. Besides my wonderful marriage, I delivered my two kids at home without the help of any medications and I continued my professional career. My life was easy and beautiful.

In October of 2012, however, both of my parents passed away and less than three years later my youngest brother was kidnapped and murdered in Mexico. My world fell apart in those years. I believe that these two incidents were the ones that triggered the cancer, as my diagnosis came a few months after my brother's death, but they were not the cause. I knew I had to find the root of it. I believe that all illnesses are created by thoughts and emotion, with the latter merely being an accumulation of thoughts that you eventually believe to be true for yourself. I knew that cancer is the physical manifestation of deep hatred, one that you may not even be aware of anymore. So where was this hatred I was holding on to placed? and how could it be remedied?

I was an abused child, physically, emotionally, and sexually, no wonder I was experiencing cancer! That type of pain buries itself so deep, that you are no longer aware of it until an emotionally traumatic event happens opening the door for cancer to develop fast.

The diagnosis was confirmed, there were two tumors, one invasive and the most aggressive type of cancer: HER2. It was time to start working!

I knew that if the cause was mental, the only way to heal is mentally. Cancer is a symptom, never the cause. But I also thought that if it has already manifested in a physical form, I must work on my body too, so Chemo and Radiation were not for me. I researched and read everything I found on alternative ways to heal breast cancer. I spoke to many different people all over the globe, traveled and I did everything in my power to heal myself. I never doubted my ability to heal myself.

I punched pillows, imagining that those pillows were the aggressors, until I had no more resentment.

I started to work on forgiving all those who ever hurt me as a child. I also had to forgive my brother's assassins. It was not easy, but I did it knowing that my health depended on this.

I managed my emotions using the skills I learnt through Mental Application.

After that, I started to fill myself with love. If cancer is caused by deep hatred, which is the opposite of love, it could only be healed by true love. I said affirmations all day long and always included these in my meditations.

To my twenty-year routine practice of Transcendental Meditation, I added visualizations and affirmations from *Joe Dispenza's* online course, that I bought through Hay House.

I knew stress favors cancer, and stress is fear, so keeping myself relaxed and in a loving state would calm the stress and had to bring healing.

I decided to get rid of toxic people. And I did! When you have cancer, it means that your body is intoxicated. This means that your mind is also intoxicated. So, you have to eliminate all the toxins from your life. I followed *Dr Veronique Desaulnier's* protocol for the physical part of it.

I cut out sugar of all kinds from my diet. No more gluten for the rest of my life. Dairy too was eliminated and I followed the Food Combining Protocol.

I took many, many supplements. I still do!

I fasted several occasions over a year.

I moved back to Mexico which is where I always wanted to be.

I only talked about the cancer to very few people, the ones that I knew would support me in my decision of not going the conventional way.

Thanks to Cathy Murphy from Heal Thy Self from Dis-Ease, I found out that bouncing on a Cellerciser Rebounder may stimulate the lymphatic system. So, I bought it and loved it.

I did a colon cleanse every single day, and sometimes twice a day for a year.

After six months of following this protocol, I was feeling better than ever. I had lost thirty pounds, was full of life, and I looked younger. My hair was shiny and abundant again, my skin was radiant and young-looking. I was thriving. Nevertheless, I decided at that point to have surgery. I had a mastectomy from which I had a speedy recovery.

Within just one day I no longer felt the need for pain medications. I went home the following day after the doctor told me "You are cancer-free". They insisted on the chemo and radiation, but I never did that.

At the time I am writing this, five years later, I am sixty-four years old, alive and well and now guiding others on this beautiful path. I am also free from all fear.

Lucia Stone

Chapter 22

Healing Multiple Myeloma Through Dietary Changes

I t wasn't long after applying as crew on Thomas' yacht in Mallorca, Spain, that our whirlwind romance began. Both with similar dreams of sailing around the world, both with a sense of adventure and passion for a life at sea, we were thrown into the depths of a romance novel. Yet neither of us reckoned that our biggest challenge would be a health crisis in my birth country, New Zealand, just before a world pandemic.

At the ages of fifty-six and fifty-seven, we were fitter and healthier than most of the sailors out there, or so we thought. Unbeknown to us, in the bilges of the boat, lurked an unreachable toxic concoction of diesel and oil. A large mass of foam under our large fuel tank had absorbed spilt substances over the thirty-year lifetime of Qi, our yacht. This and other factors contributed to an accumulation of toxins in Thomas' body that eventually would show themselves as life-threatening blood cancer.

Over the winter of 2019, we flew to Thomas' home country of Germany to visit his family and to attend his work summit in Barcelona. Thomas felt a spike of pain in his upper back. Putting the twinge down to having moved awkwardly, he sought explanations and relief for a strained muscle as no amount of pain relief was working. After visiting two doctors without success, three weeks after the initial accident, we were becoming concerned as he seemed to be getting worse. Not wanting to begin any major testing or hanging out at hospitals where neither of us spoke much of the language, we waited until we returned to our base country, New Zealand.

Topped up on painkillers, we made the trip back to New Zealand and went into an emergency medical centre. The doctor did a blood test and gave new painkillers.

It was the next day that we got the call to visit our doctor as soon as possible because there was a high level of calcium in the blood. Looking up what this might mean on the internet had us horrified. 'A condition that occurs in the final stages of cancer'. The doctor was young and lacking experience, but Thomas was relieved to find that he spoke German. He came out of the consultation saying that he'd been told to come back next week to check his bloods again and had provided Thomas with even stronger painkillers. Nothing was working to relieve the pain in his upper back.

The following day, the doctor's surgery rang back and said get to the hospital as soon as possible. At the hospital, they did an x-ray, more blood tests and filled him up with morphine, then outlined their suspicions: All results and symptoms were pointing to Multiple Myeloma, a blood cancer. The x-ray revealed a crushed vertebra at T4 where cancer had caused a tumour in the bone and weakened it.

Twenty-four years earlier, I'd completed a three-year course on Nature Cure Naturopathy. Thomas and I often butted heads with our differing paradigms about health care and the power of healing. Still, when he was released from the hospital, we quickly modified our already vegetarian diet. I'd strayed from my true course to adapt to Thomas' diet and eating habits and the challenges of being at sea for long periods of time. Fresh produce wasn't so readily available. But now we were on land and we began having celery juice and more fruit. Thomas had given up his strong expresso and sugar. He didn't even feel like his daily beer.

Weekly injections of chemo and a concoction of steroids and other support drugs were showing various side effects; tingling feet, constipation, brain fog. But his remission came quickly and within three months the cancer indicators were extremely low. The next step in the treatment was a stem cell transplant and the haematologist began to prepare us for this, giving us a leaflet of information.

Thomas read the leaflet on the stem cell transplant and was convinced that he didn't want to go down that avenue. He was ready to listen.

115

Searching for alternatives for this type of cancer gave up no sources until an advertisement for Chris Beat Cancer came up on my Facebook feed. He was offering free viewing of the ten videos in his series.

We watched the whole series and, even though it was promoting a different philosophy to my own, it was close enough and Thomas was interested. He began choosing different aspects of the approach Chris was advocating and he began implementing these, plus the Budwig Muesli ingredients of quark, a type of cottage cheese and some organic flaxseed oil. Thomas began interval fasting, eating his Budwig Muesli after his celery juice and his plate of fruit between 11am-12pm. I would juice carrots, beetroot, ginger, turmeric, lemons and apples and he would drink this throughout the afternoon. Our evening meal was a large salad, but this soon changed to include a small portion of something cooked. We were finished eating by 7pm.

We'd removed any processed foods and other cheeses from our diet. Thomas was still getting his chemo shots and the arrangements were going ahead for the stem cell transplant – right in the middle of the Covid lockdown. It was time to make the big decision. Leave the allopathic approach behind altogether and just go natural or try and do both? Being told that he would be on a type of chemo for the rest of his life, or as long as the public funding would last, was the deciding factor. We're sailors. We need to be free, and staying in the harbour wasn't an option for spending our days together.

After three months, Thomas was beginning to feel himself again as the after-effects of the chemo were fading. He had a short three day fast, picked up his mild exercise routine shortly after and hasn't looked back.

Monthly blood tests have revealed that his cancer indicators have dropped to the point that they are undetectable and Thomas has been completely drug and supplement free for nine months now (January 2021). We continue the diet with some modifications. The carrot juicing has ceased and the amount of Budwig muesli has been decreased. Thomas is feeling healthier than he has in years and the best part is, his mojo is back. We're loving life, sailing around the waters of New Zealand and hiking in this beautiful country until the world opens again. We won't turn our back on cancer. We'll continue our natural lifestyle forever.

Gaylyn's philosophy on health, Nature Cure, prescribes that the body will heal itself when the causes of disease are removed and the organism is placed within the eight conditions required for life. This is as long as the body has the energy available and hasn't reached the point of no return. The body can take a lot and will usually respond well to a natural regime such as this, but there's no way to measure how much energy the body has.

The eight conditions for life include:
1. Air – fresh, clean air breathed deep into the bottom of the lungs
2. Diet – a diet of natural foods between the hours of 12pm - 8pm. 50% -fruit, 35% vegetables, 10% carbs, 5% protein. All plant-based with the exception of the quark in the Budwig Muesli. 80% raw foods. No refined sugar, low carbs, no processed foods, no coffee or caffeinated teas, no alcohol
3. Spinal Care – to enable the nerve energy to reach the organs
4. Rest – good sleep, resting after meals and physiological rest in the form of fasting when a fever is present
5. Water – clean, filtered water that is energised in the sun
6. Mental Poise – feeling confident, full of hope and gratitude. Spiritual growth.
7. Exercise – in the right portion to suit the body's condition. Strength, flexibility and aerobic
8. Sunshine – a morning sun bath taking in the cleansing and invigorating power of the sun

These conditions require more detail and methods surrounding their application. Gaylyn offers educational programs on these that can be found on her website.

Along with the physical regime, mental poise and belief that Thomas would undoubtedly heal were adopted from the beginning. We believe in the healing power of love and received it from friends all over the world.

Gaylyn Morgan and Thomas Runte

On our boat SY Qi (pronounced Chi), currently in New Zealand

Chapter 23

Natural Healing of Stage Three Vaginal Cancer

I n May 2001, I was diagnosed with stage three vaginal cancer and immediate surgery was recommended because I was told that my life was in grave danger. I wasn't sure this was the best course of action for me as I believed that this cancer had been growing for some time. There was no rush to do anything until I'd had a chance to process this information, and then decide how I was going to deal with it. I had a strong belief in cause and effect so I was curious to find out what had contributed to the cancer, and particularly in the genital area. I believe that if I'm powerful enough to create an illness/disease, then I'm powerful enough to uncreate/heal it using the tools and strategies that I had learned over the last fifteen years.

First of all, I prayed for the help I was going to need to heal my condition and waited for the guidance/signs to come to me. It was fascinating to watch where the assistance came from but I trusted and followed the information I received. I had been attuned to Reiki one and two for some time, so I was able to send healing to the whole situation which hopefully would reveal the root cause.

From the late 80's I had a keen interest in the body/mind/spirit connection and became an avid reader of many personal development, spiritual and metaphysical books eg. *"You Can Heal Your Life"* by Louise L Hay. The probable causes of cancer are:- "Deep hurt, longstanding resentment, deep secret or grief eating away at the self, carrying hatreds. What's the use." That's interesting I thought but had no idea what it related to, but believing in Louise's philosophies, I adopted her affirmations for this which are - "I lovingly forgive and release all of the past. I choose to fill my world with joy. I love and approve of myself." I set about using these straight away.

A Holistic Doctor in Brisbane had been recommended so I made an appointment to see him as well. He tested me for everything to see what my body needed to regain good health. My energy and immune systems were quite low and some important elements in my body were almost depleted. He prescribed a very high protein diet and I had to eliminate sugar, white processed foods, coffee etc and I was given lots of vitamins and protein drinks to restore my body's health. So, home I went with all this 'stuff' and started my new health regime.

Each time I checked in with the Doctor in Brisbane, my health was continuing to improve. I got another letter from my Doctor in Bundaberg, very similar to the first one (three in total), to say that my life was in grave danger and I needed to have the surgery as soon as possible. I wrote to this Doctor to say that I had decided I would not be going ahead with the surgery and that I would be using alternative methods to heal myself.

There was never a time that I had any fear – hard to explain, or doubted, that I would be able to heal this cancerous lesion. At this time, I had a dream where I was shown that my bottom was pink and clear just like a baby's bottom so I knew that it was healed in spirit and all I had to do was find out how to dissolve the lesion in the physical, mental and emotional bodies.

After four months of seeing the Doctor in Brisbane, he told me that my health was 'A-OK' but the cancer lesion had grown by about fifteen percent and it was spreading up inside my vagina as well. He wanted to book me in for surgery then, but as I left his clinic, I told him that I still wasn't convinced that I needed to have an operation. I found it interesting that even though my physical body was perfectly healthy, the cancer was still growing.

On my four-and-a-half-hour drive back to Bundaberg, the message came to me that I had not found the root cause that had created this condition. What a 'light bulb' moment!! Then I got really excited and knew that there was more work to do but I felt that I was getting closer to the mark.

During a Reiki treatment, my practitioner asked me what happened when I was about five or six. She had been given some insights about what the issue was but was unable to tell me as I needed to "find" out for myself. I prayed for help as I consciously had no idea what it was all about. It obviously was buried deep and had been forgotten. After more loving prompting, I was given a name and that's when I knew we were onto something from the reactions in my body. I continued praying and through divine guidance, I was given the understanding that I had been sexually molested when I was about five years old. Then I really started to sob as I knew deep down inside that this was the truth for me. With this new knowledge, I had something to work with and maybe I had found the core wound that had started the cancerous lesion nearly fifty years ago.

So, the next level of healing began. Forgiveness played a huge part in the actions that I took next. I thought about all my sexual experiences, and partners, and forgave each and every one of them. I forgave myself for the bad choices I had made regarding my sexuality and also the beliefs I had 'made up' while growing up, regarding intimacy between couples, and my need to say 'Yes' to whatever was asked of me.

To my amazement, within days, I could feel that the lesion was reducing in size but I dared not look as I don't think I could really believe it. Within a week, the lesion had completely gone – OH! What a Feeling! With a strong belief and focused intent, it took six months to dissolve and heal. It just proves that as we create our dis-eases through our stored emotions – like hurt, guilt, anger, shame, resentment and unworthiness we can reverse the effects and bring about healing by letting these go through forgiveness.

It was the proudest day of my life. I was so excited when I realized that the cancer was gone, that I had believed in myself and my choices till the end. We are powerful beings and I now believe that anything is possible.

So, my recommendations are: -

Do your own research.

Trust yourself as you know yourself better than anyone.

Find the solutions, whether it's food, therapies or treatment, that feel right for you.

Don't rush into any decisions when you're feeling overwhelmed.

"The past is what influenced my life's choices,

Now my new choices continue to create a better future"

Kaylene Hay

Author of

For the LOVE of SELF The Proven Tools and Strategies for Healing my Life

Colitis

"The most powerful relationship you will ever have is the relationship with yourself"

Steve Maraboli

Chapter 24

Ulcerative Colitis; A Journey from Victim to Magician

O k, so when this health story started, I was only a few years into my 'journey' to understand how the universe works. I had read 'The Holographic Universe' by Michael Talbot and had started reading around Taoism, giving me insight and understanding of the mind and its power. But I wasn't yet at the point of accepting that I had the power to be healthy, that I was born to be healthy, or that bad health was in any way related to mindset, beliefs, diet and all of those important things. I COULD have noticed, but one only sees the truth when one is ready.

Looking back, there was a lot of evidence about health reflecting the inner world. I had, for example, been in a previous long-term relationship and from the start of it, I'd suffered from terrible tonsillitis. This recurred savagely and often over all the nine years together, continuing as bad throats even after my tonsils were removed. It ended magically, immediately that she and I broke up! So yeah, I was still believing that the body was a kind of machine and that it would go wrong sometimes and that doctors would fix it.

The health condition I want to talk about here, though, is ulcerative colitis, where the wall of the colon becomes sore, inflamed, painful, bleeding, sometimes losing control. As anyone who has had this 'symptom' will know, it is not a great thing. It is embarrassing because of frequency and urgency of toilet visits needed, and it is debilitating because of blood loss, internal inflammation, secondary infection, terrible pain and all that stuff.

So, when I first got a few little parts of the 'symptom' of this condition, ironically just some constipation and pain, I was living in France and went to French doctors. But, for a second opinion, to make sure that I did the right thing, I also flew over to the UK a couple times and saw UK doctors too.

I had suffered from digestive problems over a period of a few years previously. These were upper digestive problems, from my oesophagus, stomach and upper intestines, characterised by soreness, inflammation, sometimes feeling something was in the way of food being swallowed, creating too much saliva etc. I underwent an oesophagoscopy, a camera popped through my nose and down to my stomach to have a look. I was then given pharmaceutical medications, anti-acids, Gaviscon and all that parcel of chemicals to try and modify stomach acid, reflux and the like. To be fair, I think one of the doctors at that time said 'avoid stress', the ONLY comment I had from any conventional medical personnel either then or related to the colitis - around twelve in total - that wasn't advising on treatments to 'fix' a bodily behaviour.

Because of the colitis, I had a colonoscopy, a camera in at the other end! The upshot of all the consultations I had in France and the UK, was a diagnostic and prognostic endpoint that went along the lines of, 'We don't know what causes colitis. Treatment is first anti-inflammatories, next steroids, finally surgery.'

I would like to mention again - and it seems incredible to me now! - that none of the doctors I saw in either country talked to me about diet, about belief, about biome (the healthy bacteria in one's gut that are also linked to brain health) or about anything other than pills and the surgeon's knife. Nor did ANY of them have any thought that the condition could be cured or reversed. And actually, when you think about it, one of the many background beliefs of "conventional" medicine is that a chronic condition only gets worse. Another is that when the body misbehaves, drugs and surgery are the go-to options.

Well, so there I was with a gloomy prognosis, a debilitating and embarrassing condition and a repeat prescription for VERY expensive pills (costing the NHS something like £100 per month I think) and, to be honest, I felt very disempowered. At best I sometimes felt that determination to 'fight' that you hear about from, for example, cancer sufferers. But fighting is not something really related to health, is it? And if you're fighting yourself or the world, what then?

I took my pills and suffered the symptoms and thought unpleasant thoughts about the future and, steadily, things got worse. They got worse to the point that blood loss made me stop being vegetarian and try to eat lots of red meat (often microwaved ready meals if I was feeling too weak to cook). At the same time, I was working in the pub industry and, in the course of my work, doing endless shots of tequila and other spirits, plus I was a parent to young children. Only determination kept me functioning. In my love life, I was flitting from one toxic relationship to another.

BUT all the time I was doing something else. I was spending more time with healers and energy workers and acupuncturists. I was starting to learn about the mind and training as a Master in Neuro-Linguistic Programming (NLP), hypnotherapist and a range of therapy techniques. I was understanding more and more about things like quantum physics and the ways in which we - literally - shape and manifest our reality, on a physical level.

At some point, I reached a decision. I remembered the medical advice and said 'fuck that', I threw my pills away and immediately felt better. I decided that I could be and was responsible for my own health and could manifest the health I wanted.

Fast forward about seventeen years from the first 'colitis' diagnosis and I look back on that person I was then with love and compassion and understanding. No wonder he felt lost. He came from a system that had brought him up from birth to believe that there was a finite universe 'out there', a world that was 'true' that he couldn't change, and that at some point he would be a victim of its workings.

He was taught to believe that doctors knew best about health and that the body could let you down. He was vaccinated with all that was given at the time he was young and fed and injected with enough antibiotics during the repeated tonsilitis episodes to wipe out and unbalance healthy bacteria and many bodily harmonies. And he certainly hadn't spotted that things like relationship choices or diet or any of the other things going on were to do with that most basic of all health and wellbeing factors, loving relationship with self and with the environment.

I am not yet quite symptom free but very nearly. I eat a beautiful organic, mostly vegetable diet because I know that this is a way to send love into my body. I only choose and accept relationships or life situations if they are beautiful and healthy and empower me. I give thanks for all the blessings of my life. And I accept responsibility for all that I am and all that happens to me. Being a victim in any way has been left behind forever because I realised this was significant in my suffering. I am in control. Which is what I was born to be.

Finally, I am lucky enough to help many people to reach the mindset of personal love and empowerment in my breakthrough therapy work. You can read about some of the ideas that feed into that work in my eBook 'Your Life Does Not Exist... (...so have another one any time you like)'

Patrick Cave

Chapter 25

Ulcerative Colitis or Not?

I was working and living a very stressful lifestyle. Corporate America was getting the best of me. I was working in healthcare and expected to go above and beyond. I was slowly killing my body, working like a maniac. I always say that the sickest people are in healthcare and/or the medical field because their jobs are to put others first.

The irony is even though I was working in western medicine, I absolutely did not practice or necessarily agree with all of its terms because it uses orthodox methods of diagnosing disease and does not look at the big picture. I had always been into alternative, holistic medicine and was doing my best to take care of myself under those harsh conditions.

All those things played a huge role in my mood and health. One day I decided that I couldn't take the negative people and high stress, any more and I quit my job. As I was taking time to rest, restore and recalibrate, I started diving deep into yoga, meditation and Ayurveda. These practices had always been a part of my life, but they got pushed back due to my lifestyle. All of the weight lifted off of my shoulders and I became much happier.

About four months after I quit my job, I began to have slight diarrhoea, which I blew off. Then, that turned into diarrhoea plus blood in my stool. At that point, I knew something was very wrong but still didn't do anything. I just didn't want to think about it and for some reason, I thought it would go away.

I ended up diagnosing myself with ulcerative colitis because of the extensive knowledge I had in my previous career. This is a digestive disorder, which is also known as inflammatory bowel disease. It's considered to be an autoimmune disease, which means the immune system attacks the colon. In my case, my immune system didn't recognize the difference between good and bad bacteria in the gut. Thus, attacking everything and causing a huge imbalance in my large intestines.

I couldn't believe it because my diet was extremely clean, at that time, I was a hardcore vegan and I was slowly transitioning into becoming a raw vegan. I did not eat gluten, soy, sugar, dairy, eggs, processed foods and I didn't eat out. Every meal I prepared myself, so I knew exactly what was going into my body. My diet was and still is significant to me. I was only eating whole foods like fruits, vegetables, grains and legumes.

As time progressed, I lost a lot of weight, became weak and fatigued. In addition, I experienced rectal pain, nutrition deficiency, became highly anemic and was cold all of the time due to the blood loss. There were times when I couldn't get out of bed because I was so weak. Some days I was able to function without any physical attributes and then there were times when I was able to be mobile, but definitely felt the energy drain from my body with every step. I was so fragile and didn't have the stamina to keep a job, so I was unemployed but I knew I could reverse all dis-ease within my body.

I was fortunate to have a healthcare/medical, plant-based culinary and yoga/meditation background. With that being said I still had to do my homework and relearn a lot about the body and how all the systemic functions work together. I researched all I could on the internet.

I knew that dis-ease developed in the gut because our gut is our second brain, so that's where I started. I became my own healthcare advocate. I knew I could heal myself naturally and that is what I wanted to do. First thing I did was get a colonoscopy because I needed an official diagnosis, so I could understand where exactly the problem was in my large intestines. For me to understand the western medicine approach was important, so then I could take that treatment plan and transmute it into alternative means.

Next, I taught myself Ayurveda because it is the oldest health system that uses a natural approach to healing. Ayurveda helped me tremendously because it was individualized to me and only me, verses conventional medicine, which relies heavily on big pharma and surgery. Healing for me was a mind, body and soul effort, a holistic approach, to go to the root cause of the imbalance.

Through Ayurveda, I found out that my diet was not serving me and was making me even sicker. Even though I was eating pure foods, it was the way I was approaching it that did not work for my body and this dis-ease. As Hippocrates said, "Let food be thy medicine and medicine be thy food," but you have to understand your specific body type.

Going on the elimination and anti-inflammatory diet was key. This allowed me to figure out what was agreeing with me and what was not. As I was already eating clean, alkaline and plant-based, the main change I needed to make was to eat all warm and cooked foods for my digestion to truly heal. Again, this was specific to my body type or dosha as they call it in Ayurveda.

I took immune-boosting herbs, spices and supplements to build up my immunity and adaptogens to reduce the stress I had put onto my physical body. Some of my favorite herbs are chamomile, boswellia, tulsi and ashwagandha. I took NAC to repair the damaged tissue in the intestines. Another supplement I started taking was spore-based probiotics to help with my gut microbiome. And lastly, I took a liquid iron supplement to help with my strength, energy and rebuild my red blood cells because I was losing a lot of blood.

I chose to go to an Acupuncturist because I didn't have an Ayurvedic clinic near me. I learned about lymphatic drainage and how this is beneficial for the body. Exercise was also a part of my daily routine because I knew I had to sweat out the toxins and release all the stagnation my body had stored. The exercise was easy some days and harder the others because I didn't always have the physical strength or energy, as ulcerative colitis is very exhausting. I made sure I moved my body when I could and rested when I needed to.

Meditation, yoga and breathwork helped a lot with the stress. Showing my gratitude for everything I was thankful for in life, lead to more abundance. I took the time to appreciate all the things I did have because like attracts like; it's the law of attraction. The main thing that I needed to get control over was my stress levels and following my true path. I hadn't been living my highest purpose, which also led to the imbalance in my body.

For me, spirituality became a huge component when it came to reversing all my symptoms and healing myself. Labels (diagnoses) are overrated, so I decided not to attach myself to the negativity of my diagnosis because thoughts are very powerful. What you think is what you become. I incorporated positive affirmations and mantras into my life every day. My top three favorites are: I am healthy, I am healed, and every cell in my body is thriving at its highest vibration.

People thought I was crazy and wanted me to buy into the system, but I knew it didn't align with my values; I knew I had a higher calling. I listened to that voice in the depths of my soul. I know for a fact that our bodies are self-healing, smart and speak to us all the time. I became more intuitive and went inward to figure out what my body was trying to communicate.

Healing wasn't easy and it took me years to get the situation under control. I never gave up because I believed in myself, had faith and knew this was the right decision. Every day was different and I had to honor my body on where it was at. It took time, but I stayed patient and consistent. Funny thing is, years later I found out by an Ayurvedic doctor that I was actually misdiagnosed and I did not have true ulcerative colitis. My body was going through a shock because of the high stressed lifestyle I was living. All in all, healing naturally is absolutely possible. I was kind to myself and my body. It's the best feeling in the whole entire world when you do what is considered, the impossible. It's a miracle and no money in the world can buy that priceless feeling.

Karina Melissa

Chapter 26

Healing Colitis to Become a Health Coach

My story starts in 2004 when I became sick, very suddenly whilst on holiday in France. Although I now know my story really started soon after I was born, (I shall come back to that later).

I was twenty-seven, healthy and newly married. Yet out of nowhere, I experienced horrendous gut symptoms including heavy bleeding, pain and exhaustion. It took several months of tests, examinations and scans to receive my diagnosis of Colitis. A form of Inflammatory Bowel Disease which affects the large intestine.

Initially, I was relieved for an answer, thinking "now that I know what it is, it will be ok". I was expecting to be given a cure to 'make it better', allowing me to go back to the life I had before. However, I was naive. Rather than a cure, I was told I had an "incurable disease" and it would be "lifelong". This was not how I had imagined my life panning out. It took time to adjust to this news, I went through spells of sadness and despair at this new life that had been thrust upon me. I was prescribed various medications, which changed depending on how my body responded. Amongst those medications were Pentasa (Mesalamine) and Prednisolone, various forms of both, which I would take from dawn to dusk.

With so much medication in my body, I doubted I would be able to start a family, something that I previously took for granted.

I accepted the medication route but as years passed, I became anxious at my reliance on drugs and the risk that my body may stop responding to them. Other Colitis patients often need increasingly more extreme treatments and oftentimes, life-changing surgery. I felt like I was dangling over a ravine on a fraying rope, not knowing when the rope would snap.

This was when my mindset shifted. I started to investigate why I was sick and how it started. Yes, I had a grandmother who had a bowel issue, but was this enough for me to be in this predicament? I needed to know more and opened my mind to who could help me. I came across Kinesiology, a therapy which focused on my whole body, a body which I had taken for granted for years. With the help of this therapist, I discovered specific foods were depleting my energy and that my body had become out of balance. It was fascinating. Armed with this advice I adjusted my diet to remove foods that were causing inflammation in my body. I stopped eating dairy, wheat, soy, sulphites and some other foods that I couldn't tolerate. This fuelled me to look deeper and I introduced several supplements, again, on the advice of my Kinesiologist.

The most important change at this point was a feeling of empowerment. No longer did I feel that this chronic disease was out of my control, the outcome wasn't purely in the hands of medical specialists, I had to take the responsibility for my health

Throughout recovery, I ensured that I was exercising. I felt the benefit of moving my body in whatever way was achievable, according to my symptoms. I still feel that exercise is hugely important today to help support my gut health, digestion and overall wellbeing.

When I cut out harmful foods from my diet, I naturally started making healthier choices and increased plant-based foods on a daily basis. I was eating many more vegetables than ever before to increase the nutrients in my body and support my large intestine. This definitely made a difference.

Fast forward some years, I sustained these changes and gave birth to my first baby, we relocated to another part of the UK to convert a barn (with no previous building experience)!

Admittedly, moving to a building site, weeks before I was due to give birth to our second son was not the best plan, but I had been feeling incredibly well with no symptoms and this was a great opportunity for our little family....

Soon after giving birth, I became ill with mastitis, an emergency appointment saw me heading home with a course of antibiotics, which I gratefully took to relieve the hell of the infection! However, within days my health came crashing down - bleeding heavily and depression - I had plummeted back into a Colitis flare. I was heartbroken, I had no idea that antibiotics could do me such harm, as I had no real knowledge about how my gut worked.

Horrendous forms of medication were prescribed and I sobbed daily at administering the treatment which left me in pain and feeling nauseous. With a newborn, a toddler and a building site to contend with I was in the worst place I had ever been.

But every cloud has a silver lining. My desperate situation led me to meet another therapist to bridge the gap now that I was far away from my Kinesiologist. I am so grateful for the day that I met the Craniosacral therapist that I still see to this day. Her decades of knowledge and immense wisdom taught me that there was so much more to know about my body. With her expertise and support, I headed back into good health once more.

"So, is this the end of your journey?" No, it was some years later that, once again, my health hit a block. I had a feeling that stress wasn't doing my health any favours but I never 'switched off' and thought I 'thrived' on stress. Juggling children, a home and a career with travel around the UK - I was at breaking point. The climax occurred at the office when, again, I was in the midst of symptoms but something was different, I couldn't think straight and I silently broke down in front of my computer. The rest is a blur but I somehow made it home, to bed whilst my body went through a prolonged panic attack.

That was my last day in the office and the end of my career. My body had hit its limit of what I could push it to and it flicked the switch

I couldn't go on like this. At forty years old I had to decide what I was doing with my life. My Craniosacral therapist recommended I train in nutrition to understand my body better, which I did (pretty daunting when I hadn't studied since I was eighteen)! Two nutrition qualifications later I felt much more in tune with my gut and how food is medicine. I introduced probiotics and these had an incredible impact on my remaining symptoms, so much so that all medications stopped at that point.

I also found Functional Medicine (an approach that focuses on identifying and addressing the root cause of disease) and it blew my mind that there was a medical model which married up with the work I had been doing for myself since my twenties.

Once again, I was a student but this time to become a Health Coach. I learnt about the root cause of disease, self-care and how to recover from disease by changing our lifestyle. I also studied stress and emotions and how these two factors can impact health.

It was from my experience of stress that Emotional Freedom Technique (EFT) came into my world and I loved it immediately. I trained to become a Practitioner to understand how to address negative emotion, stress and trauma to enable me to manage my life with a stress-free approach

So, here I am today, healthy, strong, symptom and medication free and feeling better than I have felt since I was young.

When did my story really start? My health did not simply plummet in 2004. I have learnt that my health was declining, slowly and silently, since I was born. Chronic Disease doesn't just appear by chance or bad luck. It accumulates within our body, over time.

I believe that being bottle-fed from birth, years of antibiotics for chronic ear infections, being a terribly fussy eater, acne medication, fifteen years of the Contraceptive Pill (linked to Colitis), alongside a stressful career and never, ever, listening to my body......that's why I got sick, these are my 'root causes'.

After many years of sickness and forty years of life, I found my purpose. I knew that I wanted to help others realise their own potential for healing. To put the power back in their hands to allow great health to happen, maybe this is why I had to be sick.

We must never take our health for granted. We must also believe there is always hope for recovery. Our health needs to be managed throughout our life and we can embrace every lesson we learn along the way.

Rachel Turner

Gut Health

"All disease begins in the gut"

Hippocrates

.

Chapter 27

Healing My Gut Health Led to Healing Ulcerative Colitis, Candida and Carpal Tunnel

As a complementary health practitioner for over thirty years, I look back at where I started from on my journey to health and wellness.

I started my career on the other side of medicine as a Research and Development Chemist in the Pharmaceutical industry, working on prescription-only drugs. I enjoyed my job and even though I smoked, I was young, had a good diet and I felt well.

When I became pregnant, I gave up smoking, gave up social drinking and stopped working with noxious chemicals. Then I became ill with ulcerative colitis, a very unpleasant condition where the lower part of the large intestine becomes ulcerated leading to diarrhoea and bleeding – a lot! Before this, I'd rarely had sick days, but now I was off work quite a lot, spending much of my time on the loo. Going out was a complete nightmare. My social life virtually came to a halt – which is something that usually doesn't happen until after the birth! Stress made it worse and having it made me stressed.

Seeing the doctor and consultants meant that I was offered medication which as an expectant mum I really didn't want. I was also quite bloated and towards the end of the pregnancy, I developed carpal tunnel syndrome, which got much worse after my son was born. It started out as pins and needles in my hands during the night and progressed to pain and tingling in my hands, wrists and arms at night and during the day, which meant I really struggled to pick up my son at times. I eventually had operations on both hands (separately) which really helped, although it would return temporarily if I did anything repetitive with my hands, knitting, typing or gardening for example. Then when I had my daughter, it returned, not as badly as the first time but enough to be painful.

After I had my son, I started Yoga classes and discovered that the centre where they were held was putting on an Alternative Living Day. I must be honest; it was the cookery class that appealed the most! However, I also went along to a talk on Reflexology. I remember Pam who gave the talk, asking the lady she was demonstrating on if she had a bad back and was it around the T3 area – yes it was! Well, I was very intrigued, but hugely sceptical due to my science background. I went home and tried pressing various points on my husband's feet. His big toes (the head reflexes) were very painful and he suffered from migraines - could there be something in this?

I found a health magazine at the newsagent and borrowed the only book on reflexology from the library. This of course was well before the internet and complementary medicine was definitely on the fringe then. These only strengthened my interest, so I enrolled on a reflexology course and qualified when I was pregnant with my daughter. I used reflexology on my children throughout their childhood, they had very few ailments and no medication.

I had also continued delving into alternative health magazines and books, which although thin on the ground, increased as time went on. From the information in these, I stopped eating the sugary foods and started taking acidophilus (good bacteria for the gut, which are now well recognised for the role they play in gut health) and slowly my gut started to improve.

I also cut out eating bread (which I loved), because of the yeast and the wheat, both of which can be detrimental to gut health. Again, I noticed improvements in my health.

It was around this time that I discovered kinesiology, and whilst training, testing confirmed that I had issues with sugar, wheat and mercury too. A kinesiology technique helped my body to eliminate the stored mercury.

I also noticed that whilst writing assignments up on the computer, this too could upset my bowels. Simple things like running my central meridian before and after spending time on the computer really helped. The central meridian is like a storage battery for the whole meridian system and the electromagnetic field of the computer can easily affect it. Other kinesiology techniques helped to heal my gut permanently. I can't remember the last time I had any problems, which is fantastic when you consider that for many people with ulcerative colitis the outcome is often a partial removal of the colon.

The carpal tunnel which came back when I had my daughter, has also disappeared, due in part to better gut health but also from taking a multi-B vitamin. The B vitamins are great for stress and anxiety and vitamin B6, in particular, is good for carpal tunnel.

In the beginning, I felt like I was fumbling in the dark as there wasn't much information available. Now it is so much easier, we can find out virtually anything within minutes through Google.

With the benefit of hindsight, I can see how it all began. I was raising my blood sugar levels artificially by smoking cigarettes, which of course stopped when I was pregnant. I then found another way to boost them with toast and marmalade, cakes, biscuits and I was pretty much addicted to cheesecake! This sugar overload combined with the hormonal changes due to pregnancy were ideal conditions for candida to flourish in the large intestine.

As I was overloading on wheat, my gut was unable to process it efficiently and so it became an irritant. That and the candida caused my gut to overreact, by eliminating constantly and destroying the lining, leading to ulceration. This of course was very stressful, which again added to the problem.

The key things for me, were to stop eating sugary foods, eat healthily, take probiotics, balance my meridians (which also helps the related organs) and use stress relief and other kinesiology techniques. These were all instrumental in getting my health and vitality back. I now enjoy eating a wide variety of foods, including bread!

Having been in complementary health for over thirty years, I have seen many clients presenting with a wide variety of problems and often there are underlying gut issues that need addressing.

I always give my clients self-help techniques they can use at home every day to support and maintain their health improvements, self-care is so important. Good health is our own responsibility.

This led me to write a book during lockdown for people who want to make improvements to their health and wellbeing, but have limited time.

I hope this inspires you to start your own health journey.

Linda Hoyland

Author of

Five Minute Fast Fixes – quick and easy ways to improve your health and wellbeing

Chapter 28

Healing My Gut to Heal My Life

Growing up I was the kid who always had a cold or flu. As a baby, my mum and I made multiple visits to the emergency room to seek relief from my painful ear infections. The recurring ear infections were of significant concern and it was recommended that my tonsils be removed, even though they form a part of the body's immune system.

I was four years old when I had my tonsillectomy. This surgery started a cycle where I ended up sick with a cold, flu, or throat infection roughly every ten to fourteen days, leading to at least five rounds of antibiotics each year between the ages of four to eleven. I remember looking forward to going to the doctor solely because it meant that I was going to get banana flavoured medicine.

In 2005, I went overseas to New Zealand and while preparing for the trip down I headed to the pharmacy to get everything that I was going to need for a three-month stay. Antihistamines, anti-inflammatories, an inhaler, antacids, daytime and night-time cold and flu medications, birth control, steroid cream, and more. A friend saw this bag once and said, 'dang, you have the whole pharmacy in there'. It was a lot of over-the-counter medications and, unfortunately, at nineteen, I required something almost daily.

I met my now-husband in 2008 while living in Melbourne, Australia. I remember feeling insulted the day he said to me, 'you are sick all the time.' I wasn't sick all the time. Or was I? He pointed out that I was making trips to the pharmacy at least once every two weeks to pick up something to help me function.

In March of 2014, I had a miscarriage ten weeks into my pregnancy that led me into depression. Then I developed eczema, that covered my whole body, including my face. I went to my family doctor to see what tests were available to figure out what was going on. I was given a steroid cream and told to get an allergy appointment.

In May of 2014, I began noticing eczema flare-ups after eating certain foods. I started listing these, to remind myself to avoid them. It got so bad, the skin on my forearms became cracked and weeping. I went back to the doctor to ask for help and was given a prescription for antibiotics because I was at risk of secondary infection. I went into hiding during this stage.

I was working as a nanny and only went out to public playgrounds and the occasional grocery store because I was ashamed of how my skin looked covered in eczema. I would turn around if I saw someone I knew, so as not to bump into them and I cancelled a lot of plans that summer.

After a particularly hard few weeks of painful and itchy, eczema-cracked skin, waking me up in the night, I went back to the doctor. I was struggling to sleep, lying awake on the couch watching shows, while searching on my phone for people who had a similar story to mine. The doctor told me to take an antihistamine before bed to help prevent itching from the beginning.

In July 2014, while driving out to a family reunion I was massaging my neck and shoulders to relieve ache and tension and I discovered three lumps in my neck. I made an appointment with a doctor as soon as I got home. During that appointment, I was told they could remove the lumps and test them for cancer. Can you test before cutting? I asked thinking about the permanent, easily visible scars this procedure would leave, already knowing how badly I felt when people stared at my eczema.

'No, we cut now and test later'. I went home very discouraged. After three months of going back and forth to the doctor, I had not received any answers or lasting relief. The list of foods to avoid was getting longer and the eczema flare-ups were constant. In early August of that year, I had reached my breaking point. I went back to the doctor determined to get a solution.

I explained my constant eczema flare-ups and how my skin was so thin that it easily split and bled. I was offered steroid cream and told to take antihistamines to manage the itch. I shared how the list of foods that triggered flare-ups was over seventy items long. I was told to avoid anything that irritated the eczema. I explained my weight was fifteen pounds less than an average adult weight and how my hair was falling out, that I couldn't sleep at night and I was exhausted and how incredibly frustrated I was because everything changed over the course of a few months.

I was then told that what was going on with me was 'bad, but it wasn't bad enough to do any further 'testing or investigating'. I went home so defeated and angry. Soon thereafter, during a particularly bad eczema outbreak that had swollen my eyes half shut I was putting laundry away when my husband came home from work. He came up to see me and when I turned around, he sat down and said, 'What can we do to help you'? I broke down, I had gone to the doctor multiple times. What else was there to do?

I don't remember what sparked the idea to go back to my homeopathic doctor. At my appointment with her for the first time, I felt heard. Based on previous reactions to candida cleanses she said it sounded like I had candida overgrowth. Candida overgrowth can cause a leaky gut and a leaky gut can be linked to chronic eczema. I left with anti-candida herbs, soothing drink mixes for my digestive tract, and a limited diet plan.

I was gluten, dairy, sugar, and alcohol-free. Anything that caused inflammation was cut out because it could stop the healing process. I drank a litre of bone broth a day for a month and ate mainly vegetables and gluten-free grains.

The restricted diet wasn't hard as I had already been living with a long list of what I needed to stay away from. The herbs were hard to choke down, and the candida die-off reaction made me want to quit taking them, but I started to feel better a week later. After another couple of visits and new remedies, I was no longer having recurring skin issues, my weight stabilized and my hair was no longer falling out.

As my digestive tract started to heal, I was able to eat more foods that had previously created an eczema flare-up. I remember feeling empowered when I threw that list in the garbage, I could now eat and not feel nervous. Within a month I started to feel like myself again. My skin was getting stronger and thicker and I could make plans to see family and friends without worrying I would have to later cancel.

Also, the lumps in my neck had disappeared. After we helped my gut, we started working on helping my liver. I had been taking something over the counter for around twelve years almost daily and my liver needed a break. I wasn't back to my normal self, but then I wasn't sure what my normal was. I had been sick every ten to fourteen days since I could remember, and I needed to focus on ways to help build my immune system.

It has been six years since this health crisis. I went from thinking I was going to have to survive on air and water to now being able to eat anything. I am a healthy weight and my hair is long and lush. I have two healthy boys and I get sick maybe twice per year.

Healing comes in all different forms, always push for answers when you don't feel heard. If advice and recommendations don't resonate with you, find another opinion. You matter, your health matters. Treat food as medicine, self-care starts in the kitchen.

Ashley Pharazyn,

Gut health coach

Chapter 29

Healing Our Gut Healed Our Bodies, From Hashimoto's and Autism to Vibrant Health

Ten years ago, I found out I was pregnant with my first child. I was ecstatic until I received a phone call from my physician telling me that my pregnancy hormones were not going up and that I could lose my pregnancy. I had blood work done and was found to have pregnancy-induced hypothyroidism. I was immediately prescribed Levothyroxine and was able to carry my first born to term. It turned out that a lifetime of eating the Standard American Diet (S.A.D.) and environmental, as well as emotional stresses had triggered an autoimmune disease.

Following my son's birth, I struggled with all of the symptoms of Hashimoto's disease. I was gaining weight even though I was dieting and barely eating. I had a puffy face and eyes, severe light sensitivity, terrible anxiety, I was cold all the time, I had extremely dry and flaky skin and hair, joint pain, brain fog, digestive issues, constipation, headaches and even depression. You name it, I had it.

My hair loss was so severe that my doctor even prescribed Rogaine treatment for women (which didn't work). I was fatigued all the time and just miserable. I felt that my body was against me, and in a way that is what autoimmune diseases feel like because your own body is attacking itself.

I was so severely hypothyroid that my physician referred me to an endocrinologist. I thought that seeing a specialist would surely help and I would soon find solace from the misery of thyroid disease. Sadly, her medical advice didn't differ. Apparently, the only way I was advised to manage my symptoms was to take medication for the remainder of my life.

Meanwhile, my son was two years old, experiencing severe facial rashes and eczema and wasn't developing at the typical pace. He was walking on his toes, flapping his arms, not making eye contact, and hadn't started speaking yet. He was diagnosed with Autism Spectrum Disorder.

I was a single mom, working full-time and feeling like my whole world was falling apart and my health was deteriorating. I had always been an action-oriented, problem solver so I went back to school part-time while working full-time and became a certified holistic nutritionist in the hope that I would be able to take control of my son's and my own health matters without the need to be medicated for life.

Armed with nutritional and scientific knowledge, I changed my son's diet to dairy-free and gluten-free. I also put him on an extreme supplement regime. His body was starved of nutrients and after two weeks on the diet, he started speaking and a few short months later he stopped flapping his arms and walking on his toes. Today, he is ten years old and loves creating YouTube videos.

As for myself, I made a lot of changes. I was so desperate, and I was getting told by my doctors that I would need to be on medication for the rest of my life. I changed my diet to a no sugar, no gluten, no dairy, no caffeine, no alcohol and no processed foods diet. I found out that sugar and gluten were especially harmful to the thyroid as they attacked the thyroid gland and were some of the main culprits in my reoccurring flare-ups.

It is believed that hypothyroidism is the symptom and inflammation is the actual disease. So, to treat the symptom (hypothyroidism) you must reduce inflammation in the body because the immune system is over-stressed and exhausted. The overall aim of the treatment is to relax the immune system long enough to end the chronic inflammation.

My diet consisted of anti-inflammatory foods such as a lot of healthy fats from avocados, nuts and seeds, ghee, olive oil and coconut oil, salmon and sardines. I focused on consuming organic produce whenever possible and organic meats and eggs, grass-fed beef and wild fish. I included fermented foods like sauerkraut, kimchi and kombucha with almost every meal of the day to help restore my gut health. I made fresh organic vegetables the main attraction in most of my meals but omitted nightshade vegetables like tomatoes, white potatoes and eggplants for their inflammatory properties. Through the changes in my diet, I was able to heal my gut so that it would be able to absorb vitamins and minerals from the foods I ate as well as the supplements I took.

The supplements I took to replace the nutrients that my body needed more of were zinc, B complex, Vitamin B12, magnesium, vitamin D, selenium, and iron.

As for my lifestyle changes, I had to find ways to reduce stress in my daily life. What worked for me was going for long walks in nature. It gave me a chance to connect to nature and felt like a walking meditation as I would appreciate the simplicity of Mother Nature. Practicing yoga helped me find my breath and taught me how to breathe deeply and with purpose which allowed my body to deliver oxygen properly to all the cells. Journaling helped exude the hustle and bustle of thoughts in my mind onto paper and was a great tool for self-reflection.

My immune system was misbehaving, and I made the decision to make drastic changes to help it heal. I embarked on an anti-inflammatory lifestyle for almost a year. Through these changes to my diet, exercise and stress management routines I have been able to get off all medication and stay off all medication for years.

My mission is to help other busy individuals struggling with weight, stress, and immune system disorders to find sustainable solutions in their everyday lives. The key to healing is not found in going through extreme dietary and lifestyle changes but rather to learn how to make manageable changes that all contribute to optimal health. After all, it took years to get to a place of "dis-ease", it didn't happen overnight and it will take time to heal as well.

Jowita "JoJo" Mohr

Certified Holistic Nutritionist
Yoga Teacher, Health Coach
Food Allergy Mom
Autoimmune Disease Warrior

"I aim to educate and empower naturally minded individuals looking to manage their health, weight and immune systems through healing exercises, healing foods and healing lifestyle changes."

Chapter 30

Multiple Health Problems from Candida Healed with Nutrition

My story began in 2010 when I was in my early thirties. I had just birthed my third and last child. I had two babies (twenty months apart) and a six-year-old. Since I was tandem breastfeeding, I expected my periods to take an extended vacation. How wrong I was; they started up within two months of giving birth. What was troubling is that they came back with a vengeance. They were heavy, painful, and lasted for weeks.

I was not sure if the change to my cycle was due to having two babies back-to-back, or if it was because I was not getting enough nutrition for myself due to breastfeeding both babies. Either way, I started delving deeper into nutrition. I had already stopped dairy because my second child had a severe dairy allergy when he was born. Since he was breastfed, I had to alter my diet to eliminate allergens.

As time went on, I began having more and more challenges with my body. I started getting migraines three to five times per week. I also had digestive issues, eczema, anxiety, depression, my hair started falling out, and I still had periods from hell. I hadn't even hit forty yet and I felt like I was falling apart. At that point, I decided to try seeing someone for nutrition response testing.

She gave me a list of foods I was reacting to, as well as a bag full of supplements meant to support my body while I healed. I stopped eating gluten right away and began looking for replacements for some of the other things. Quick trips through the drive-thru for dinners on busy days were over. I began reading labels on everything. I read anything I could get my hands on about autoimmune responses to foods and as I changed my diet, I started feeling better. That is until I hit a plateau.

I stopped making progress and stayed neutral for a while before feeling sick again. I developed a horrible rash under both arms, raised, red, and painful. I blamed my deodorant (mostly the aluminum in it) and started trying every natural brand on the market. It didn't really help much until I began to see a correlation between certain (sugary) foods I was eating and the rash appearing. I also started getting an instant headache every time I had a glass of wine. I was frustrated and angry. I was sick and tired of being sick and tired. I saw so many doctors and had so many invasive and painful tests. I was told over and over there was nothing wrong with me, it was all in my head, and I should take antidepressants and exercise.

I went back to researching everything I could until I started seeing a connection between all my symptoms. My research began to point to severe candida overgrowth. I read up on all the triggering foods; grains, dairy, alcohol, sugar, eggs, vinegars (which are in every condiment), and even some fruits were contributing to candida overgrowth. I planned on how to eliminate them, then I did, all at once.

I mostly just ate protein and vegetables. It was really hard on me because I had to make everything from scratch, including condiments like ketchup and salad dressing. Not only was I eating differently than the meals I was cooking for my family but I also had to visit an Amish farm for all of my meat because I was reacting to the grains that conventional meat farmers feed their livestock. I had withdrawals and detox symptoms like crazy. When candida cells die, they give off a nasty toxin that makes you feel horrible and give you terrible breath. But I did it for six straight months and I felt amazing!

Soon after, I joined an MLM company to make a little side money. I was raising kids, home-schooling, and running the house but we needed the extra income. I attended an online party that a friend was having, and I was talked into joining by the consultant. I'm not one for selling for these companies, but something told me it was the right choice to start selling tea. One of her networking suggestions was to offer a refreshment bar for someone hosting an event so that people could try the product and fall in love with it. I knew someone that owned a meditation studio about an hour away and coincidentally she was holding a class on the energetic frequency of foods. The thought of being in that environment with my ethically sourced tea and allergen-free treats sounded perfect!

After arriving and setting up, I listened to the presentation. I couldn't believe what I was hearing. This woman that was presenting had a story almost exactly like mine! I was absolutely flabbergasted and spoke to her after the presentation. She told me more about her own health journey and how she healed herself and her son and ended up getting certified in health coaching because of it. I had never heard of a health coach, but it resonated so deeply in my heart that I knew that's what I was supposed to do.

Since that day, I have become an internationally certified health coach, a reiki master, and began my own company to serve others and teach them how to heal themselves. Because I listened to that feeling you get when you know you're on the right path, I now have a life I thought was only a fantasy. I LOVE what I do. I find so much joy in sharing my own journey with others so that it can help them heal as well.

Thank you for reading my story. I hope it inspires you to take control of your own health and start living your best life right now!

Tina Hakala

Reiki Master
Internationally Certified Health Coach
Sacred Roots Holistic, LLC.
Host of the podcast The Foul-Mouthed Goddess

Hormones

"The body is a self-healing organism, so it's really about clearing things out of the way so the body can heal itself "

Barbara Brennan

Chapter 31

Reversing Type Two Diabetes

When I first started dating my husband Steven, I knew he was overweight and a type 2 diabetic, managing his condition with the usual pharmaceutical medications (Metformin, Gemfibrozil). He was diagnosed as a type two diabetic about five years before we met. On our first date, we went for a walk around the old town of my home city and I was worried when I saw how slowly he was walking and how quickly he got tired.

As our relationship progressed and we decided to live together I told him I wanted to try to help him to reverse his diabetes. 'It is impossible' he said at first, but I had already witnessed my dad's diabetes being reversed and knew diabetes reversal was achievable.

My dad had been a diabetic for about twenty years when I took both of my parents to a health centre for a wellness check-up. To get all of our health back on track, we all did a detox together, eating nothing but vegetables for about three weeks.

Everyone benefited from it and my dad's condition visibly changed over the course of a couple of days. On just the second day of the detox, his blood sugar level stabilised and he no longer required his pharmaceutical medication. This was all done with the doctor's assistance.

My dad didn't have any side effects from the detox and new way of eating and he felt better each day. He also lost about 10 kilograms. Dad did well for several months until he slowly went back to his old eating habits. Unfortunately, that brought his diabetes back.

Wanting a permanent diabetes reversal for my future husband, I needed to make him accustomed to the way I was now eating. After my previous cancer diagnosis, I researched food, nutrition and lifestyle for the first time. I started understanding how big an influence our daily decisions have on our overall health.

My new eating habits were primarily focused on cancer prevention, but I knew it was really an illness prevention way of eating. Besides, if we were going to live together happily ever after, I couldn't really eat any other way than a whole food plant-based diet. I believe that changing my diet and lifestyle is what has kept me cancer-free for nine years now.

Every day I would prepare healthy meals for us and explain nutrition to Steven. It was important that he understood why we were eating this way. Steven also took the initiative and started cooking plant-based meals himself.

I saw this process as an opportunity for Steven to understand that diabetes is reversible. I hoped that after a couple of months we would do a vegetable detox, as I did with my parents. The plan was to get Steven used to healthy eating, then do the detox and follow on with healthy eating.

Something unexpected happened instead. Steven had his regular diabetic check-up after only four months of our living together and changing his eating habits when his doctor told him he no longer needed to take his diabetic or cholesterol medication any more. Since this happened, he has had a diabetic check-up every six months for the last two years and he is now considered diabetes free.

By simply eating a plant-based diet he cured diabetes. Had he not changed his diet and lifestyle he would be on medication for the rest of his life. We didn't even have to do the vegetable detox.

Steven also lost 14 kg and his cholesterol reduced from being very high to healthy levels. He is now active, plays tennis, cycles and we go for long mountain walks and Steven proposed to me on the top of a mountain he thought he would never climb.

I wanted to share Steven's journey to raise awareness that type two diabetes is reversible. You just have to ensure you lead the healthiest life possible by eating natural, wholesome foods and being active.

To date, I have been researching diets, nutrition and lifestyle for almost ten years. This information fascinates me. We can control so many health conditions and problems just with changes to our daily habits.

Mila Bromley

Chapter 32

Healing Me Takes Time, But Starting the Journey Is the Hardest Part

---

'm Laurie, a forty-five year old mum from Scotland. I'm a self-employed Holistic Therapist and have been practising for nine years. I've always struggled with my weight, and I've been a serial yo-yo dieter most of my life. My healthy food choices were salads, sweets and stodgy comfort foods. I had no idea how this contributed to my health issues over the years and I'm not completely healed, but well on my way. This is my story.

Over the years, the conditions I suffered with were never actually diagnosed until adulthood. I had suffered through my teens bouncing from one type of prescribed medication to another, simply just trying to dull down the pain of heavy ten-day periods, cramps and headaches.

I struggled every three weeks to even step foot out of bed and when I did, I could barely walk across the room because I could not straighten my back and every time I moved, I could feel the blood draining from my body. I formed an extremely bitter relationship with my hormones and reproductive system. By the age of fourteen, I was quite an angry person.

My teens were horrendous, but adulthood wasn't to be much better. Following the birth of my daughter via caesarean section and further investigations, it was discovered that I had endometriosis, an awful condition that affects the reproductive system of women.

Endometriosis causes the womb tissue to grow in other parts of the body and currently, the only treatment is pain relief, hormone replacement therapy or surgery to remove the tissue. Surgery, however, creates adhesions, the sticking together of tissues, which causes more pain and discomfort.

In addition to endometriosis, I also suffered from many health issues; persistent urine infections, candida (vaginal thrush), pelvic adhesions and internal scarring from the caesarean section, stomach ulcers, gallstones, a cyst on my kidney, the menopause, a hiatus hernia and I had a disc removed from my lower back, leaving me with nerve damage. I also may have Irritable Bowel Syndrome or diverticulitis. All these health issues come with a range of symptoms that cause me a variety of problems, as you can imagine.

My own healing journey began in 2017 when I discovered meditation. Initially, my meditations involved a guide, talking me through visualisations and scripted journeys, but further research led me to sound frequencies and vibrations. I started tuning in daily to frequency healing with binaural beats and solfeggio frequencies and was blown away with the results.

I was altering the frequencies of my brain and this was having an amazing effect on my outside world as well. My husband even commented on how calm and patient I was and I felt more peaceful in myself. I realised then that what I was thinking, I was creating in my reality. I found out that this is the Law of Attraction and it was unfolding before my eyes, opening up a whole can of worms for me to deal with and heal.

After a few months of gaining this mental clarity, confidence and strength I introduced the mineral moringa olefiera to my daily routine. Moringa contains over ninety vitamins, minerals, antioxidants and anti-inflammatories. It contains vital proteins and omegas, and although it looks awful, it's very drinkable and tasty.

A friend introduced this to me through her network marketing company and as much as I didn't want to be involved in network marketing, the product actually did work for me. I was able to come off all my medications within the first week of introducing this super green smoothie to my diet. It was amazing.

My hot flushes from menopause stopped, the inflammation in my colon/intestine reduced, the heartburn stopped and the pain in my joints and muscles has eased off. I even have more energy to do more of the things I love and although I still have the odd flare up, though I'm very well aware that it's because of my own mindset, or in fact, I've missed a few days of my moringa or meditation.

My journey is exactly that, it's a journey...my destination is unknown and I will simply continue on my path of self-discovery, learning and sharing with others as I go. It's far from over. My healing is an ongoing journey because I still have the conditioning to work through. Triggers keep popping up on repeat which sets me back with my eating habits.

On a normal day to day basis, my diet isn't perfect, it never has been, but I know without moringa in my body I would be so much worse. So, until I successfully deal with the mental health issues, the majority of my days are without pain/discomfort, but I still have what I call flare-ups. These are around every two to three months and last for about a week, mostly on the right-hand side of my body, which I know is connected to masculine energy/influences.

It's like self-sabotage. When life is going well, I tend to look for things to pick fault in, my mindset shifts and then the poor eating habits or avoiding meditation kicks in. As I said, I'm still work in progress, but I hope that by sharing my journey, it will help others.

I decided to become a therapist myself because of the healing my body had undergone and I wanted to practice what I preached to my clients.

Laurie Graham

Chapter 33

Balancing Your Hormones

How did the Wild Yam Cream enter my life?

When looking for something, that something often falls into your lap. About eight years ago, I was talking to a lady that drove our school bus about problems with hormones. She advised me to try some hormone balancing cream. I thought why not and used about a quarter of a teaspoon of the cream daily, which equated to two tubes over the month.

The cream was a mixture of Mexican Wild Yam (Dioscorea Villosa), Chaste Berry (Vitex Angus-Castus), Ylang Ylang, Chamomile, Rose Geranium and Lavender essential oils. These oils are known to have the ability to relieve some of the many symptoms of hormonal imbalances and are regarded as safe, without any known side effects. Being a cream, it is easily be absorbed by the body.

After the first two months, my heavy bleeding was almost back to normal. My gynaecologist had scheduled me to have a hysterectomy which I now no longer needed, so I cancelled my appointment.

During my journey to wellness through a non-pharmaceutical, non-surgical time, I heard about the side effects of toxic ingredients in everyday products, from Phillip Day (a researcher from the UK), who had come to Australia for health events, as well as Dr Peter Dingle (a researcher from Perth in Western Australia) and Chris Woollams, (founder of Integrative Canceractive charity) who also spoke in Australia at health events.

After hearing from them how toxic many products are because of the chemical ingredients they contain, I changed my personal care and home care products over to safe ones they had recommended. These newly found ones would not disrupt my hormones as my previous products had.

I also learnt how important the liver is with hormonal issues and as a detoxifying filter. I took a course of the supplement 'Liver Health', which included ingredients such as milk thistle, vitamins, and plant extracts, to support my liver.

Today I am much healthier. I continue to use the balancing cream daily as well as take colloidal minerals and green powders daily for healthy, strong bones and body. I listened to Dr John Lee on a CD that was given to me and realised that the continued use of the wild yam cream would help to keep my bones strong, as I grew older.

Colloidal Minerals are suspended in a liquid form and are absorbed into my body quickly and easily. Dr Linus Pauling said that every disease and illness can be traced back to a lack of mineral. He won two Nobel prizes for his studies.

So why are micro minerals lacking? Early harvesting, transporting, storage, cooking and canning etc. Mineral deficient soils lead to mineral deficient plants. Mineral deficient plants lead to a mineral deficient body. Our bodies cannot manufacturer micro minerals, so where do we get them from?

I also mix a green powder supplement with the colloidal mineral each day. It has 28 different greens and supports a healthy digestive system through active enzymes and promotes detoxification.

Phillip Day, Dr Peter Dingle and Chris Woollams all say that diseases occur in an acidic body. These Green powders alkalise my body to help prevent illness and disease. I will be forever grateful to our local bus driver who put me onto this way of healthy, clean living.

Carolyn Evans

Books I found useful:

'Oestrogen –the killer in our midst' by Chris Woollams

'Dangerous Beauty' by Peter Dingle

'From Hormone Hell to Hormone Heaven' by Eva Torner

'Cancer –why we are still dying to know the truth' by Phillip Day

'Health Wars' by Phillip Day

Chapter 34

A Stranger in My Own Skin

This is how I felt after I had been diagnosed with an 'emotional breakdown' due to a severe hormone imbalance as I was approaching the Menopause, known as the Peri Menopausal stage.

This was a place I could never envisage being in, although maybe I should have had an inkling. I remember my Mum being in a very bad way and thinking she was going completely mad when she was going through the 'change'.

The signs were subtle at first, with my body shape changing. This was soon going to be spiralling out of control, only to see me engulfed with fear, not knowing how the hell I was going to get back to my 'normal' self.

Shaking uncontrollably, retching with fear and not being able to stop my mind, it was like an out of control hamster on a wheel. What was happening to me and how or who was going to help me to get back on track? Unable to even get the washing out, I was not able to work, couldn't drive myself, didn't want to be on my own, yet too much company was tiring.

Sleep was a stranger and all I wanted was someone to put me to sleep for a few weeks and then wake me up and I'd be ok, or possibly wave a magic wand and hey presto, all would be well. If it was that easy, then we would have no lessons to learn and I truly believe that I was given this, so I could go on and help others who are suffering in the same way, without the use of pharmaceutical drugs.

The trip to the Doctors was a waste of time. I said I think I am approaching the menopause and they pooh-poohed it, saying they would do the Follicle Stimulating Hormone test (FSH) but informed me that they doubted my hormones were imbalanced. I was offered anti-depressants and counselling, then sent home without a care. I had told them I didn't want anti-depressants and asked if they had read the contraindications on the leaflet that comes with these drugs....suicidal thoughts etc....God who makes this up!

The key to my recovery lay within myself. All I needed to do was unlock it, as after all 'Our bodies write their own prescription'. Firstly, and most importantly I had to find some calmness, so I could reconnect with the wisdom that lies within.

A friend who used to come and visit me suggested that I saw a Hypnotherapist and even though I was in a deep, dark hole, something felt right about this suggestion. The appointment was made and my lovely partner took the time off work to take me. I left with a cassette tape (yes it was a few years ago). On one side was a guided meditation and on the other side was music that held subliminal messages, which help to reprogramme the mind.

I was at the beginning and started to feel the subtle change in myself. After another couple of sessions, I felt in a calmer space. I wasn't out of the woods but it felt as if someone had pruned the trees to let some light in.

I looked into the effects of a hormone imbalance brought about by the onset of the Menopause. I was now looking for Progesterone.

My ever loyal taxi driver took me to the health food shop and I purchased some Progesterone, I remember this day vividly, it was a Monday and after just one dose, I could feel the dark cloud that had engulfed me for weeks shifting and I thought OMG this is working...footnote here, the blood tests said that my hormones were fine....I rest my case!

I can only say my hormones were completely 'out to lunch' and as our hormones are our messengers it doesn't take much to send them out of kilt. As my progesterone was very low, I did take the recommended dosage for a few days but, listening to my body, I quickly realised that too much would tip me back out of balance.

I used to hold the bottle of progesterone and ask my inner wisdom if I needed this today. If I felt a very strong YES then I would go ahead but if not, then I would leave it till the next day and ask again. I also purchased some Oestrogen and, on some days, it was that that was needed...Lord knows what would have happened to me if I had been lured into taking Hormone Replacement Therapy (HRT), equal amounts of Progesterone, Oestrogen and Testosterone...how can that work and are we all made aware that once you stop HRT the symptoms return?

We are all unique and therefore our Menopause will be unique to us as well. What is going to work for one will not necessarily work for another. It is a journey of discovery.

Our hormones are chemicals therefore, putting any unnatural chemicals into and onto our body by way of food, body lotions, shampoo and other products, had to be addressed. This has made me very aware of the chemicals we constantly smoother our bodies in and ingest, really unaware of the effects they are having on our very being.

Over the past few months, it has been made apparent that we also can have genetic diseases that are running through our bodies, unaware of the damage it is doing to ourselves.

For very many years I have had several sebaceous cysts, mainly on my head (luckily, I have a good mane of hair to cover them up). I got up quickly one day and hit one of them on the corner of a low ceiling, which caused it to burst and become infected. A friend of mine suggested a visit to a homeopathic toxicologist...she unearthed traces of Brucellosis that can affect hormones. I believe that this would have been inherited from my Mum's side of the family, with her having such a terrible Menopause too.

This journey of healing myself was not always easy but by looking for the signs within myself, I have learnt to listen to my body and mind. It doesn't lie.

It was much more than Progesterone that helped my recovery but the Progesterone was my starting point. I then used Bach flower remedies, meditation, eating healthily, exercise, being kind to myself and being outside, on my healing journey until the end of my

Menopause. It has been an adventure. There were highs and lows but I came out other side without the aid of pharmaceuticals.

Susan Horwell

Author of

A Stranger in My Own Skin, authored in my former name of Susan Irwin
Note: There are some references in my book that are no longer relevant i.e., blogs and email address.

Chapter 35

My Life with PCOS

Poly-Cystic Ovarian Syndrome (PCOS) is a big title that can wreak havoc with your life.

As a young girl I was very active and slim then puberty hit. I was still very active but I put on weight and developed an eating disorder to try to stay slim. My time of the month was terrible, if it decided to make an appearance. I had terrible cramps, bloating, mood swings, and a very heavy flow. I suffered with depression out of nowhere and it would be gone as fast as it arrived.

When I reached nineteen things really changed. I broke out in severe acne, up until that time I never had so much as a pimple so it took a toll on my self-esteem. I also started to gain weight fast. I started going to the gym for two hours a day and I would eat very tiny meals or not at all. I managed to lose about twenty-five pounds before my body stopped losing weight.

At twenty-one, I was married and I had gained enough weight that I was now right around two hundred pounds. I still had acne but I decided I wanted to find out what was going on with my period and my mom had thought that going on the pill would help not only my period but the acne.

The doctor told me that I had PCOS and he gave me a rough explanation as to what it was. He told me that if I wanted children that I should start now because it may not be possible in the future. I was married eight months when I got pregnant with my first child. I was about nine weeks along when I miscarried her twin. I didn't know at that point that there were twins until I hemorrhaged and passed one of the babies.

Outside of high blood pressure, the pregnancy was normal. I went two weeks overdue and then went into labor. I spent four days laboring with her at home until I went to the hospital and they helped it along with medication.

My daughter was three when I decided that I wanted another baby. We tried for six months to have a baby but nothing worked. Because the doctor knew I had PCOS, he gave me Clomid to help the process. It was horrible, the ovulation was so painful but thankfully it worked and in the first month of using it I was pregnant.

Outside of high blood pressure, this pregnancy was uneventful. Again, I went two weeks over my due date but instead of waiting, the doctor induced me. Surprisingly, when my second child was three months old, I got pregnant again. I remember just laughing and feeling so blessed. There again I had high blood pressure and he was induced after I went two weeks overdue.

Things to know with PCOS, you have larger than average babies. My first weighed 8lb 9oz, my second was 9lb 10oz, and my third was 10lb 5oz.

I was not able to breastfeed my babies; I barely had enough milk and I just didn't produce it. This is actually very common in women with PCOS. It has to do with oxytocin, this is the hormone needed not only to create breastmilk but also to go into labor, remember all of my labors had to be induced.

Fast forward a few years and I am now in my early thirties. I am obese, I weigh 258lbs. I crave carbs all day long and I have a terrible time controlling the urges to eat. I am depressed and I get diagnosed with Rheumatoid Arthritis. I haven't had a period in a year.

A friend convinced me that I need to go and have a checkup and she refers me to the practice that she goes to. This time the doctor orders blood work, a glucose test (the syrupy drink), and an ultrasound. She found what they didn't know about when I was in my twenties.

The ultrasound showed that I have the textbook PCOS ovaries, a bit larger than walnuts with cysts around the ovaries like a pearl necklace. My glucose test showed that I was insulin resistant. The blood work showed that I had a slow thyroid, high cholesterol, and high triglycerides. I also had high blood pressure. At this point in life, the only thing I didn't have was acne and hair loss.

The first thing that happened was I was placed on a lot of medications; every symptom got a pill but blood pressure got two pills. I was also sent to a dietician to learn how to live with my symptoms.

I remember spending an entire afternoon with the dietician learning how to eat. She taught me the standard PCOS meal plan and that was what was needed at the time. I was able to lose 20lbs on it but I needed to do more.

Fast forward a year and I had researched enough to create my own meal plan. I was able to take off 75lbs total. This got me off of all medication with the exception of my thyroid medications. It also started my periods and for the first time in my life they were on schedule every month. I started studying herbs and learned which herbs worked for me for hot flashes, premenstrual syndrome and thyroid. They were such a big help to me.

When I turned forty-five, I decided that I wanted to help others so I enrolled at Trinity School of Natural Health and became a Master Herbalist, a Certified Nutritional Counselor, a Certified Health Specialist, and a Doctor of Naturopathy. I wanted more so I enrolled in the Holistic Health and Healing program at Kingdom University in Indiana and I have finished their Bachelors and Master's degree programs and am currently working on my PhD in Holistic Health and Healing.

Diet is the number one way to control PCOS. Women with PCOS have trouble losing weight and many women deal with both cravings and sugar withdrawal whenever they attempt to lose weight.

My eating plan at the beginning of my healing journey was very regimented but it worked. I ate three meals a day and added in two to three snacks; breakfast, mid-morning snack, lunch, afternoon snack, dinner and evening snack, if needed.

I made sure that I consumed 45 grams of carbohydrate at each meal and 15 grams of carbohydrates in each snack. This kept my blood sugar steady, eliminating cravings and carbohydrate withdrawal.

As I lost weight and the desire to eat so much, I stopped the snacks but initially kept my carbohydrate intake the same for my meals. As I lost further weight, I reduced my carbohydrate intake to 30 grams per meal. My meals now never go above 45 grams of carbohydrates, on the rare occasions that I plan on having bread or pasta.

My meals are mainly made up of vegetables and proteins. A simple meal plan that I follow and teach is a plate made up of at least 75% vegetables and the remaining percentage either protein or starch. This can be started after weaning off carbohydrates.

I made sure to exercise every day. Walking has always been my "go-to", so I started with a ten-minute walk after each meal, (this is great if you're crunched for time or just getting into shape). I worked up to talking an hour walk every day and created my own stretching routine.

Supplements, I make sure to take a multivitamin every day. I also keep Black Cohosh and Evening Primrose oil on hand to help with hormone balance.

Getting enough sleep and undertaking meditation has helped me to deal with life's stressors. It is important to understand that stress can lead to hormone imbalance.

PCOS is an issue that more and more women are being diagnosed with and I know for a fact that diet plays a huge role. One of my passions is teaching about PCOS and helping women take control of it. With work, it can be overcome.

Kimberly Boutelle

Author of

PCOS and Freedom: Beating Carb Addiction

Lyme

"The natural healing force within each of us is the greatest force in getting well"

Hippocrates

Chapter 36

Healing Lyme from the Inside Out

The first thirty years of my life was no picnic and filled with much adversity and trauma. I was a child of multiple divorces on both sides, experienced emotional and physical abuse, bullying, and suffered through physical imbalances from unknown allergies, constant ear infections, migraines, and viral infections.

In college, I experienced abusive and unhealthy relationships, multiple instances of sexual abuse and a severe episode of mononucleosis (glandular fever), that was misdiagnosed as lymphoma.

Little did I know, my immune system was undergoing way more stress and I was progressively getting sicker. With symptoms such as extreme muscle and joint pain, leaky gut, IBS-D (irritable bowel), migraines, brain fog, tinnitus, neuropathy and insomnia, among many others, I knew there was something seriously wrong.

I saw specialists for every symptom and was given about ten different prescription medications for symptom management. I quickly realized that none of these helped and actually gave me more problems to deal with. I felt like no one was listening to me and I wasn't getting the support I wanted or needed. My body felt so debilitated and yet disconnected and I was losing trust in everyone around me, including myself.

During a job, I fainted for the first time in my life. This became a routine experience which hospitalized me about once a month for a few months. A microbiologist friend checked my blood and discovered I had "Stage four" Lyme disease and needed help right away before permanent damage and coinfections persisted. To my dismay, conventional doctors told me that it was incurable and I would be on even more medications the remainder of my life. That was the start of my holistic health healing journey.

I met with a Lyme specialist and immediately dove into a variety of naturopathic health protocols consisting of bioenergetic sprays, auricular therapy and a very strict diet of organic whole foods, no dairy, no processed foods or sugar, no pork or red meat, no gluten and drinking lots of water. The start of this was rough as I had discouraging Herxheimer (detoxing) reactions. But within six months of commitment, I saw and felt a major difference. I realized that when I invested in myself and was patient with the process, I saw results.

I started working again but still did not feel quite right. The science geek and humanitarian in me wanted to learn more and see what else I could do to compliment my current routine and support me not only physically but emotionally, mentally and spiritually too.

By divine intervention, I attended my first essential oil class and everything started to awaken within me. The aroma of these oils was unlike anything I had ever experienced as it touched me on an energetic level and raised my vibration almost instantly. The teachers of the class were open and welcoming and shared how the oils had led to their healing.

I started on the recommended protocol of essential oils and essential oil supplements for Lyme and autoimmune support and felt a deep shift almost immediately. Not being the best pill taker, I was a little hesitant to dive into the nutritional supplements, but once I did, I knew I was hooked for life. Like many others, it was the game changer and I would be doing you a disservice if I disregarded the power of quality supplements. I believe the combination is what truly gave my body what it needed to function optimally and I've continued with the routine ever since.

With all that is available to us in the health industry, it can be tricky and confusing knowing what products (or even foods) are safe and most supportive of our bodies. Speaking from experience, quality, sourcing, third party testing, purity, sustainability and transparency are all factors to consider before putting something on, in or around your sacred body. Synthetic components and adulteration can add more toxicity and slow down your body's healing process drastically. Doing my own due diligence and then personally experiencing the difference was like sunshine reaching the darkest part of a valley. This inspired my family and I to reduce our toxic load by eliminating synthetic chemicals, artificial fragrances and toxic ingredients around the house and with our personal care products. These simple changes can take excess stress off the body and help to yield amazing results.

I am happy to report that my most recent health scans show that the Lyme disease is no longer detected in my system. Something that conventional doctors said is "incurable" is in fact gone. I am a firm believer that your body is capable of healing itself and having natural, safe and effective tools helps to facilitate your body and expedite the healing process. It's also empowering, grants peace of mind and allows you to feel prepared with a first line of defence and a proactive lifestyle daily.

One thing I always share with others who are wanting to overcome health challenges and imbalances with holistic and natural tools is to do your own research, listen to your body and be patient with the process. It can take months or even years to heal the body from years of toxicity and poor habits. The journey is highly rewarding and will lead to greatly improved quality of life.

First things first, get to the root of what is going on. Many times, conventional testing and doctors are not looking at the whole body for answers but rather focusing on one or two symptoms. I found a company that uses bioenergetic DNA scans that gives an extensive report including stress levels, food and environmental sensitivities, general categories of resonating toxins, balancing remedies, as well as hormonal and nutritional imbalances. This report answered so many questions for me and is still a company I rely on for health updates to track my progress. Once you get the answers then you will receive suggestions to help get you on the track to healing, including essential oils and diet.

Be mindful of your eating habits. Get into a spiritual practice like meditation (I highly recommend following Dr Joe Dispenza's work), yoga, journaling, and prayer. I commit at least thirty minutes each day for reflection and spiritual practice and it can really impact mindset and emotional health which directly correlates to physical health. Also, make time for self-care and activities that bring you joy. The body and mind can heal much faster when in an elevated vibration. You are capable of more than you may realize and you also don't need to do it all alone. It's ok to ask for help and guidance when needed and reach out to people who will lift you up and hold you accountable.

The challenges I have faced throughout my life influenced who I am and gave me purpose. My mom, my mentors and my essential oil community are a huge part of the strength and healing I have gained over the years. I am so grateful for them and for the confidence and empowerment I have with my own health and lifestyle as well as being able to help others feel the same for themselves and their families whether it be emotionally, physically, mentally, spiritually or financially.

Thank you for taking the time to read my story. I hope it inspires you in taking the next steps to the freedom, health and happiness you deserve.

Melissa Marson

Chapter 37

Healing Lyme

I t was like hell ensued overnight. I went from high functioning, working for myself sixty hours plus a week, running five miles a day, gardening, socializing, living a wonderful life with my fiancée of six years, to a completely different life.

I went out to celebrate a friend's birthday and woke up the following morning as if I'd had a lobotomy. It felt like a constant panic attack and I couldn't remember how to cook. Not only that but I couldn't read a book or watch television and everything was overstimulating.

I started having dystonic reactions, tics, tremors, akathisia, severe orthostatic intolerance and went to see my doctor. I was put on Klonopin, which stopped a lot of my symptoms and allowed me to sleep. At that point, I hadn't slept for two weeks.

As I got sicker, I thought it was just the Klonopin. After one month, the doctor dramatically reduced my dose. It was like going cold turkey from the drug and I had a stroke, at twenty-eight years old. I had to have the dose increased back up. I spent the next two years thinking it was just the drug causing my symptoms. I tried to come off it but got sicker and sicker.

At this time, I didn't realise that my house was full of black mold. I started having seizures but they didn't show up on any of the electroencephalograms (EEG's) that I had, yet nothing stopped them. I lost the ability to eat solid food, walk and talk, at various times.

Finally, someone told me they thought I had Lyme. I was tested by my doctor and two days later, I had my answer. I cried for three days straight, thinking I had a death sentence. I then tried every treatment imaginable; Bee Venom Therapy, Myers Cocktails, Glutathione pushes, Buhner Protocol, Antibiotics, Results RNA, Parasite Cleanses, Colonics,

Enemas, Cranial Sacral Therapy, Acupuncture, various diets and many supplements. Nothing worked and generally, they all made me worse.

I had my DNA tested and things started to make sense. I couldn't detox from mold and I lived in a tent in the winter in Seattle. My lymphatic pathways were blocked so anything that moved toxins like activated charcoal would have me on the ground screaming for death feeling like I was being electrocuted alive. I got lucky and found Pekana Big 3 which allowed me to finally tolerate charcoal.

Many of my symptoms seemed like a form of encephalitis and because of this, the doctors tried to do a spinal tap, which went wrong. It took them seven attempts to get fluid out of my spinal cord. I was hospitalized for five days, by Doctor Najjar one of the top neurologists in the world. He wanted to study my seizures because he didn't know what was causing them.

Another neurologist diagnosed me with either Paediatric Autoimmune Neuropsychiatric Disorders Associated with Streptococcal Infections (PANDAS) or Paediatric Acute-onset Neuropsychiatric Syndrome (PANS) and prescribed me low dose Intravenous Immune Globulin (IVIG) at home. I almost died at all three tries because IVIG is suspended in sulphur amino acids and at low dose creates more cytokines, causing me to go into anaphylactic shock. I felt like I was losing my mind.

Finally, another doctor said that my tonsils were the worst he had ever seen and arranged for me to have them removed. This alleviated a lot of my symptoms. I then tried homeopathy, which helped and I conceived my daughter.

The day after her delivery I was given the Rhogam shot, an injection made up of antibodies. This sent me into a layer of neurological hell I cannot describe. I had to be hospitalized five days after delivering her as I could barely lift my head and I was hallucinating.

My daughter was given to my ex-boyfriend and I was sent home, where I needed around the clock, full-time care. I found TRS, a product that detoxes heavy metals. After only one spray, my brain and body calmed down. I started to get better little by little.

Two weeks after delivering my daughter, an MRI scan revealed a lesion in my brain, that wasn't there before. The report cited "drug damage". I feared that I could never be able to take care of my daughter and lost my dream of being a mother forever.

I still was sick and bedridden, having seizures and I developed cataplexy where I would randomly pass out. My symptoms list was so long I couldn't write it down if I tried. My viral load was higher than it ever had been and I had new infections from Rhogam which contains untested human plasma.

I was introduced to BioReigns products and Limitless was the first of their products that I tried. It gave me back some energy and brain function through regeneration, from BDNF peptides. After this, I used their daily CBD tincture and my seizures stopped (I am now almost four months seizure-free after years of having them sometimes for years).

Then came the game changer. A friend sent me Shilajit, a natural substance found mainly in the Himalayas, formed for centuries by the gradual decomposition of certain plants by the action of microorganisms. Everything changed. Every day, I started to feel better, my capabilities increased, my viral blood results all became the lowest I had ever seen, my blood count looked better than it did when I was in my twenties and I no longer was pre-diabetic.

I continued to get better, moved to the country and have remained stable. I am finally loving life and am totally symptom-free. I cook three meals a day, walk, run, work and clean. I can now read books, watch movies and television again. I have my personality back and I can feel love and happiness once again.

Because of my journey, I learnt to read raw genetic data for chronically ill people, to help them troubleshoot treatment, supplement and medications. I love my life now; it is beautiful on the other side.

I hope my story can give others hope that anyone can heal, it takes patience, strength and determination. Healing is not just physical but mental, emotional and spiritual too.

After six years of sheer mental and physical torture, I am me again!!

Kristina Stephenson

Chapter 38

Opening to Guidance and Becoming the Healer

My healing journey began in 2013 after an extended, overuse of antibiotics for skin issues which ruined my gut, along with working almost seventy-hour weeks, eating processed and chemical-laden foods, not prioritizing sleep, and running myself into exhaustion. My skin started erupting in cystic acne, my stomach was in knots, and I started developing food sensitivities.

I threw all prescription pills away, did some research and concluded a few things. That I had wiped out my precious microbiome - the amazing and necessary gut flora that not one doctor had told me about, and that I had a systemic candida overgrowth based on all the lovely gastro and skin symptoms I was experiencing. So, it was time to choose myself and my health.

I gave up drinking and changed my diet to whole, organic, unprocessed foods as much as possible. That alone made a huge difference for both my stomach and skin. After much confusion, fear and uncertainty, I was guided to a practitioner who did things differently. She used a unique system of kinesiology and biofeedback that was able to tell me what I was reacting to, the pathogens in my body, and the herbs and supplements to clear them. I knew there was something special to this work, rooted in energy and plants. Everything about it made sense and felt right on the deepest level. After maybe a month on a protocol that included natural antifungals, probiotics, and staying away from trigger foods, I felt myself come back to life. I got answers that I hadn't gotten from any doctor or blood test before. I learned that my symptoms were a result of an overwhelmed system. Overwhelmed with years of compounded stress, pathogens, toxins and chemicals (and later would find out runs much deeper than the physical).

Time passed on, I left one of my jobs, was sober and feeling great, had a new outlook on life, and my healing journey was the catalyst to my spiritual connection. I started practicing yoga as a way to relieve stress at the end of the day. But what it really provided for me was the ability to connect with myself, feel in to energies, and sit with emotions I had repressed for years.

I started a new job in 2014 thinking it was more aligned with my newfound beliefs and who I was becoming, but my body almost immediately started to feel like something was wrong; I felt deep pain in my joints and muscles, couldn't sleep, couldn't breathe well, experienced two panic attacks, and was overall exhausted. Eventually the pain became severe and splitting, and my mind started to freeze up on me. It went blank while looking at the computer screen at work, and there were times I was unable to respond to my co-worker and boss. I wasn't processing speech, and couldn't form sentences. I went back to the practitioner I had been seeing and her testing methods confirmed what I had guessed, and we started a protocol for Lyme Disease.

Although I was guided well by her, it held on for almost eight months until I worked to resolve it on my own. This is ultimately when spirit was asking me to find the answers within myself. To know, feel and get in touch with my inner healer. I reminded myself that anything I really wanted to figure out, I was able to.

I started to intuitively tap in, research, and eventually created my own testing process. The answers I found were confirmed by the tools this practitioner was using. It was deeper than just Lyme (borrelia). It was co-infections of babesia and bartonella, epstein barr virus, chronic strep, mold, helicobacter pylori, and others. The stress from this new job had caused these "opportunistic pathogens" to show themselves.

During this time, I had a few blood tests run. None of which showed Lyme, but an ANA titer test came back with elevated levels and was left ambiguous and undiagnosed -knowing now that it was triggered by some of these pathogens. I started cutting back my work hours little by little, and felt I was healing when away from the job, yet regressing when back to it.

One night I got home in such deep pain and sat on my yoga mat, unable to even do much yoga anymore because my knees and feet were in too much pain, and sobbed. For a short time, I thought there could be a chance that I wouldn't be able to walk without pain again, or have a normal existence. That was the first time I had a 'surrender party.' Answers came, and I knew I needed to quit my job in order to fully heal. That was semi-terrifying at the time, but I knew it was the next step and that I would figure out the rest. I developed a deep trust in the process, the timing, the universe, source, and myself.

I walked out of my last shift and felt the energy shift. I felt my body's relief. I took the time to heal, rest, and discover myself. The hypersensitive state to chemicals, pollutants and fragrances that had developed, started to resolve with the use of nano zeolite. I learned how to muscle test, so I knew exactly what herbs and supplements my body was calling for, and in what dosage. With some trial and error and a few months' time, most of my symptoms had resolved, then eventually they all did.

With my intuition as my guiding force, I now understood what I was capable of, and how I was meant to help others. Spirit sometimes has a funny way of pushing us on to our path. Sometimes we need to experience rock bottom, heart-breaking, terrifying moments in order to live again.

With my connection to source, I dove further into all alternative modalities for mental, emotional and energy healing. More time in nature, more meditation, ayurveda, herbalism, belief reprogramming, boundary work, etc. I wanted to learn everything my intuition was guiding me to. I learned a form of energy medicine that was so powerful, it felt like the missing piece to my healing puzzle. A way to release trapped emotions from the body (energetic and physical), so that the immune system was able to improve, stress cycles could complete, and wounds from the past - conscious or subconscious - were able to be released.

There was true emotional freedom that came from this work. I first did it on myself, and then realized I could do it for others. It eventually evolved into its own system, that I'm now able to teach. I never thought I would be able to do the work I do now. It's practice, patience, a shit ton of learning curves, trust, commitment, self-belief, an open mind, and resilience.

This pushed me further into emotional healing work, which meant diving into childhood trauma. I started to really recognize my triggers. So, I set an intention - "Universe, please provide me with what I need in order to resolve any layers of healing that remain" - and it certainly delivered. I was led to people, writing, and sacred plant medicines that would heal the most unseen parts of me. The inner child healing that I never knew I needed was so paramount in order for me to heal wounding and programming that formed in difficult childhood and teen years. The parts of me that felt unsafe (among many other things), were able to be seen, heard, and held by me. The process of reparenting ourselves is monumental for all of our relationships, every bit of our nervous system and emotional regulation, and for every bit of our health. The deeper we allow ourselves to go, the deeper we're able to heal.

To this day I've never taken another prescription medication since throwing out those antibiotics in 2013. I've found safer, more effective ways that would work for the long term. Life has opened up for me in ways I never once thought about. To always having the tools necessary to heal, my work in the world being a reflection of my life and inner work, traveling the country because I have a body that's able to do so, getting to play and realign when my heart guides me to (because that's become the main brain), my psychic abilities growing and opening in fascinating ways, and getting to experience the type of love I knew would be possible – that was worth working, and waiting for.

Healing precedes freedom. We can attain anything we want when we release the 'dis-ease,' wounds, patterns, programming and beliefs that impact our lives. Self-awareness that turns into self-mastery. It's the willingness to be open, receive, allow, release, process, implement, and integrate that truly heal.

Stephanie Stewart

Mental Health

*"Health is the greatest
human blessings"*

Hippocrates

Chapter 39

Healing My Emotional Trauma

My story of emotional trauma begins at a very young age. I was born in San Diego, California in 1968. I was raised in a large family, and we moved from state to state a few times every year. I changed schools frequently, always leaving my friends behind. My dad was an ex-Hell's Angel, who became a Christian. But, the gypsy spirit in him kept our family from settling down. We lived in poverty most of my childhood, but we always made the best of what we had. Our family moved to the hills of northern California in 1979. It was only a few years later that emotional trauma began setting in.

It was 1981– I was thirteen years old. I woke up to the sound of our neighbor pounding on the door of our home. I've been informed that my mom's vehicle had gone over a bluff, she had been ejected into the flooded river, and hadn't been found. Two days later, the search was called off due to winter weather. It was eighteen months later, that a fisherman found her remains several miles downstream. I didn't realize it then, but this tragedy would be the first of many. I began struggling emotionally, but still managed to get good grades through high school, and pursue my goals. Nine years had passed since losing my mom, when I lost my husband, at the age of twenty-two, just after our son was born. The internal struggle continued. Nine years later, my dad died of cancer, and I watched him as he took his last breath. Again, I was overcome with sadness, and knew that something had to change.

I went to my doctor, and she recommended depression medication, although she hadn't clinically diagnosed me with depression. I declined the medication, and tried to process the grief on my own. It was only a matter of months that I experience my first panic/anxiety attack. After my first anxiety attack, it took *effort* to keep from getting them. Thoughts of the past were enough to trigger the anxious feeling. I turned to food as a way to cope. I gained thirty pounds in a short period of time. Although I had given myself time to grieve, the anxiety and inner struggle continued.

Eight years later, my nephew committed suicide. Eight months later, his mom— my sister, passed away from cancer (2007). From the outside looking in, nobody would have known that I was struggling. I went to events, I smiled, I excelled in my work, and continued college. It was at this point that I made a *decision* to heal from the past trauma. I began actively taking steps to heal. It took a few years, but I finally felt that I was making progress. Anxiety attacks were happening less often, my emotions were stabilizing, and felt some improvement. I started taking psychology classes, to better understand my own emotions.

Six years after my sister passed away from cancer, my little brother passed away from prescribed medication. Eighteen months later (2015) my youngest sister (and best friend) passed away at the age of forty-three. In March 2020, I lost my brother. While these tragedies were heart-breaking, I found myself consciously acknowledging the tragedies I was experiencing, and not allowing my emotions to return to default. Prayer and meditation helped me to become more aware of my choice to respond, rather than to react.

Has life been tragic? Yes. But I am not a victim. I have allowed myself to grieve with each loss, but I have chosen to focus on the GOOD in my life, what I have, and who is still here. I choose not to focus on hurt, loss, or who I miss. Yes, I remember, yes, I dearly miss my family. But my focus is what I can do NOW to encourage others.

Prayer and meditation changed the way I respond to life's tragedies and challenges. I was proactive in searching for the strength, and the ability to *still* enjoy my life. For many years, my thoughts and emotions were "stuck" in a belief that I was a victim, and that these tragic events were happening *to* me. I was stuck in the default mode of just letting my mind become fixated on what wasn't working, who I no longer had in my life, and how helpless I felt. I didn't realize that I had a *choice* in how I respond. The more I understood that I can *choose* to respond with love, empathy and gratitude, the more I became empowered to live my life in a happy and healthy way, regardless of what I was experiencing in my outer world.

When I struggle with anything in my life, I pray. When I pray, I simply find a quiet place. I am still. Sometimes I speak out loud, and sometimes I speak in my mind. I simply *ask* God for strength and peace. I *talk* to Him like I would a friend, or a Father. I confirm my *belief* that I am worthy of being heard, and that my prayer has been received. And then, I wait patiently to *receive* the feeling of strength and peace in my life. Anything I want to experience in my life, I simply *ask*, *believe*, and *receive*.

Meditation is a similar practice. It has helped me in every aspect of my life. I found a quiet place in my home or in nature and initially, when I began, I used guided meditation, so I was given instruction in how to let go of incoming thoughts and mind "chatter". I also chose to sit quietly in silence, or I listened to soft meditation music. I learnt to quiet my mind, relax, let go, and dive deeper into self-awareness. Meditation is a way to connect to your higher self, your creator, and your subconsciousness.

I'm fifty-two years old, hold a Ph.D. in Holistic Medicine, I'm a published author, and speaker.
I want to encourage each of you to be the author of your own book of life! You can CHOOSE how you respond to even the most tragic of life events and situations. Meditate and pray. DECIDE who you want to be and let NOTHING stand in the way of your goals and dreams! Don't let your emotions stop you from living your life with passion and purpose!

Diana Martin-Gotcher, Ph.D.

Published Author & Speaker

Chapter 40

From Depression and Anxiety to Become a Homoeopathic Practitioner

Hi, my name is Donna, I'm fifty-six and truly blessed to be living in a beautiful area of Spain with my lovely hubby and gorgeous Breton Spaniel, Charlie.

My health problems started after a routine smear test, where I was told I had precancerous cells. I remember so clearly going for laser treatment and the smell of burning flesh, my burning flesh. It was awful. Sadly, the treatment wasn't successful so I had to go for a cone biopsy. A few days later, thinking I was alright, I decided to do some ironing. This was not one of my better ideas as I suddenly started to lose a lot of blood. Following an emergency trip back to the gynaecologist, he packed me up to stop the bleeding, however, I was left with some scarring. This caused me discomfort for many years after.

After this, it seemed my life was just a constant monthly cycle of severe sore throats, for which the doctor prescribed regular antibiotics, causing a candida infection, leading to vaginal thrush. The thrush was so severe that at times I bled.

In 1992 I believed my life had ended. It all sounds very dramatic but for me, at that time, that was how I felt. Certainly, the life I previously knew ended.

At the time, I had a very high-pressured job in sales for a tobacco company. I had moved up to Yorkshire because of my job and bought my own house. I didn't know anyone other than work colleagues, who

I only saw once a month at meetings. However, I soon settled in made very good friends, had a good social life and met my now husband.

I used to be able to jump in a car, travel anywhere in the country without a moment's hesitation and this was way before satellite navigation because my dad was an expert at directions, he knew all the roads and their numbers and could even tell you exactly how long it would take, didn't matter if you got stuck in a traffic jam, his timings were always spot on. However, one day as I was about to go out, I was gripped by absolute terror and I couldn't even leave the house.

I contacted the doctor who prescribed antidepressants. These helped somewhat and I managed to leave my house once again, to go to work.

Everything came to a head a few weeks later, I was all set to leave for work and that's when the terror struck again. My heart was racing, I was sweating profusely, my legs wouldn't move they were just like jelly and I felt as if I was going to pass out. I was having a panic attack. Although I was prescribed antidepressants, they didn't help the panic attacks.

I was forced to go back to the doctor repeatedly and each time I was just given another prescription for antidepressants and a sick note. On one occasion my usual doctor was away. Instead, I saw another doctor who gave me some relaxation tapes to listen to. I tried them because he gave them to me and I had to do something. I couldn't stay at home, in my house forever. They didn't stop the panic attacks but they certainly made them less severe. I was also referred for counselling which helped partly too.

This situation continued for many months. The company I worked for were very supportive and I shall be forever grateful for the way I was treated. Eventually though, having seen the company doctor on several occasions he told me outright that this was not the job for me and he was going to recommend that I retired. What!?!? I was twenty-eight years old, not sixty-five!!!

By this time, I had met my now husband, Steve and he was my rock throughout all of this, as were my two lovely stepchildren; something else for which I will be eternally grateful. He worked for British Telecom (BT) and they were offering very good redundancy packages. We discussed him taking redundancy and decided it was a good opportunity. He took the package and we started our own business. I was totally home office based, making life much easier. I was still having panic attacks although not so severely now.

At a business meeting one evening I met a lovely lady called Christine who was a homoeopath. I had no idea at the time what homoeopathy was. Anyway, I booked to see her and with the help of the homoeopathic process and the remedies, my life started to turn around. I became healthier, fitter and more balanced on all levels.

I became so fascinated by the whole subject of homoeopathy that I decided to do the four-year training course and following this, I did a further year of study to become registered with the Society of Homoeopaths.

Over the years I have also become a Shamballa Reiki Master, an Emotional Freedom Technique (EFT) practitioner and a Zumba instructor. I am truly passionate about health and wellbeing on all levels. There is so much we can do to improve our health and mine has certainly benefitted from all the knowledge I have gained through my study of alternative therapies.

Another blessing of working at home and not for a large company is that together, we could get a dog. I am a complete dog nut, I adore them. As a couple, our first dog was a Border Collie, Labrador cross called Oliver, who we got from the RSPCA. He was my constant companion, he followed me everywhere and would sit next to me whilst I was working. Obviously, he needed to go for walks and he was a huge help in me overcoming the panic attacks, his reassuring presence gave me the confidence to leave the house. We sadly lost him in 2003 but have been blessed with three other gorgeous fur babies since.

I still suffer from depression, some days I'm absolutely fine but others I can feel in the depth of despair, I also still get very anxious but thankfully now I have the tools in my tool bag to help me through these times without having to resort to pharmaceutical drugs.

At the age of twenty-eight and not ready to retire, I really didn't know what was going to happen to me. However, I am a huge believer in everything happens for a reason and the Law of Attraction. I was clearly on the wrong path and needed something rather drastic to set me on the right one.

Compared to many others, my story isn't particularly bad but maybe if it just helps someone to realise that if they are not heading in the right direction, it is possible to change and be happy, then I will be grateful for the opportunity to have helped.

Donna Kilgallon

Chapter 41

Micro-dosing With Psilocybin to Heal Depression and PTSD

My story starts twenty-one years ago, I was seventeen. After moving in with my boyfriend twelve months previously, following a dispute with my parents, I found myself on a slippery downward slope. You see, my boyfriend had an unpredictable violent temper and I found myself in peril more often than I care to think about.

His outbursts seemed to be getting worse and more frequent until one day I thought he was going to kill me. He had me pinned to the floor by my throat and I saw my life flash before my eyes. But something told me that it wasn't my time and I found the strength to fight back and kick him off me. I remember the look on his face, utter shock. He looked at his hands then at me then he stood up and left the room, leaving me on the floor.

Six months later, I had my first mental breakdown. I don't remember very much of it apart from rocking in the chair and the look on my boyfriend's face. I estimate it only lasted a few days and when I felt better, I made an appointment with my doctor, who was most unhelpful. I didn't like her attitude and she implied I was faking it in order to get some drugs. I told her I didn't want her drugs and left.

Almost twenty years later, I was still suffering from depression, panic attacks, nightmares and flashbacks. I was hypersensitive to violence on the television and media so avoided this as much as possible.

After a prolonged period of debilitating depression for which I was prescribed medication and regularly saw a psychiatrist, I finally decided I'd had enough. I needed to find another way to heal.

Traditional medicine and care were not improving my condition and just seemed to be washing over the real issues. I needed a solution, a permanent fix, so I started researching alternative treatments for depression and Post-Traumatic Stress Disorder (PTSD).

I found several interesting articles on the role of psychedelics as a tool in curing depression by repairing damaged neuropathways and "decalcifying" traumatic memories. The research was fascinating and I discovered that Dr James Fadiman was leading the research program which he started in the 1960s.

Dr Carhart-Harris at the imperial college London was also producing many positive results. I spent months reading the research before contacting Dr Fadiman, who advised me on micro-dosing with psilocybin. He asked if I would kindly report my results to him.

I spent the next six months weaning myself off my traditional medicines as I wanted to be clean to start my experiment with psychedelics. I then found a European website where I purchased a 15g dose of tampanensis, a psychedelic truffle more commonly known as "philosopher's stone".

When it arrived, I was so nervous about trying it. I was home alone for the first time. I was advised to take two grams every third day. It made me feel very nauseous the first time I took it and I almost vomited. After that, I didn't have any further nausea.

I felt more awake and alert but no other effects, good or bad. I carried on taking the micro-doses until the fifteen grams were finished. Four years on and I have only had two panic attacks, no relapse of depression and I feel that I have a much more positive outlook.

I went back to work, back to school and got a diploma. My life is really gaining momentum. I can now watch television and almost tolerate violent scenes. I no longer obsess about the trauma I suffered and it feels like a distant memory, which is exactly what it is.

Life is good and I'm enjoying being alive.

Rebecca Barker

Chapter 42

Emotional Health, Meditation and Healing

I am a doctor's daughter who has always relied on Western Medicine to see me through from the smallest inflictions to anything life-threatening. I was born at the clinic where my father worked and later lived the first few years of my life in an apartment upstairs where his surgery was located. From my very beginning, I was immersed in healing and it is no wonder that it has become such a fundamental part of my life.

It came as a shock in 2005 when I had to make the choice to give up my Wellness Centre to handle my newly diagnosed Type-2 diabetes. It was ridiculous that the wellness coach had now worked herself to the ground, to achieve a "lifestyle" condition. I should have paid more attention to me; my nutrition, stress levels, my lack of exercise and adequate sleep. To be honest, I was also addicted to fixing others' woes, and I often found myself thinking "who am I if I am not needed"?

My immediate reaction was to apply every tool in my toolbox in order to help myself but all was carried out in the mode of FEAR. I also tried to remember all my father had taught me but found that experiencing being sick first hand was a completely different ball game. After the diagnosis, I suffered badly due to being prescribed the wrong medication, taking me almost to the edge of entertaining suicidal thoughts. When I reached out for help from the professionals, I was merely told I just needed more time to get used to it.

The specialist kept increasing my medication to the maximum dose with the side effect that enabled me to eat up a whole roast chicken and then search for another one for dessert! That was strange as losing weight and fasting are considered the most effective strategies for reversing Diabetes. Now I became rounder and very depressed. My life had turned upside down almost overnight! I was the founder of a striving business where I got to meet many people daily and, now I was merely trying to survive in a population of one. I felt like I was trapped inside a sick body guided by an exhausted and directionless mind. In other words, I was feeling hopelessly LOST....as a doctor's daughter.

I knew I had to do something, to give myself a kind of "shock treatment", as well as to lift my spirit. I chose tap dancing as it served as a "buffer", resetting my "normality" thermostat. It worked for a while, joining the dancing troop and performing in front of an audience amused me to no ends...if only they knew!!

Gradually I felt better and more in control of my life so I purchased a treadmill, that action signalled the beginning of learning how to love and care for myself. I always had difficulty in locating that deserving "Self", but I also had the awareness that no healing could occur if I remained in this dark place.

I then took my first baby steps; ordering books, DVDs, essential oils, supplements and watched interesting videos online. This provided some small temporary lift but something was missing. It felt as if I was dragging my Spirit along instead of allowing it to lead me, so I prayed for Guidance and I enrolled and introduced myself to the online support group world. That was the miracle waiting to happen.

My two great passions in life are creative writing and connecting with people, so I very quickly became an active storyteller online. I found it very important to join only with like-minded participants in the area we are genuinely interested in and felt connected with them. Since then, not only have I made many online friendships and received support and encouragement, but this process had given birth to; my website, my blog posts, my page, as well as the opportunity to be sharing this with you right now.

As I grew stronger, I started questioning myself as to whether my emotional health might have contributed to my lack of physical health, and perhaps even co-creating my diseases. To some people, they might be horrified to see a connection between how "bad" they felt about themselves (or their situations) and how those "hopelessness and helplessness" feelings might have helped to give rise to their now diagnosed illnesses. I was very curious about this connection and also energised, as now I had something to work on. I even teased myself saying, "Oh my, how on earth can you expect to survive through such an ordeal without getting sick?" My answer to that rude question was, "NOW I WILL LOVE MYSELF BACK TO HEALTH" - with a defiant look!

I started "Cultivating Self Love" by attending my emotional health and "Creating Self Care" by giving myself permission to "let go", the two most important pillars to gain back health. I learned to respect myself, especially in the area of setting up healthy boundaries, so I would not leak my own precious energy, or suck on others' unwanted energy. I no longer needed to call in work "SICK" due to my energetic bank balance being in the red.

Now I tend to my "energetics" first so I spend twenty minutes daily meditating (twice daily is preferred). I breathe in deeply because air is generally free where I am and I enjoy observing all the silly, meaningless thoughts. I get pleasure "flicking" them off, one by one. I remind myself that I am foremost an energetic being so I deserve my attention to recharge my battery.

The idea of meditation is not to create a blank mind but to be willing to NOT entertain any surfacing thoughts so they take control, but rather gently allowing them to drift in and out. Through decades of practising Transcendental Meditation, the most precious gift was learning to let go and let God/Universe to run my life. When my mind is still and my heart open, I tend to perceive problems in a new light. Sooner or later the meditators would get their own GPS to enable them to reach that still place within and then return to it whenever needed, rebooting and recharging to our delight at the same time. The only prerequisite is to feel and trust that we are worthy to reach that centre, as all it takes is some commitment. Here is where the twins, "self-love" and "self-care" walk in. If you don't think of meditation as a gift to yourself, it is likely that you would put others and other tasks first in front of your own subtle needs.

In a nutshell, to get well, I had to accept that some changes need to be made. Stubbornly holding onto my old mindset and habits did not push me forward in a meaningful way. I needed to make a mental

SHIFT when I felt stuck, and courage only arrived when I acknowledged that the reason I was sick was because of me. On some level, I was aware that I wasn't fulfilling exactly what I was meant to do here in this lifetime.

So, getting the Diabetes diagnosis SAVED MY LIFE and CHANGED MY LIFE TO THE BETTER. Now I use this condition with the assistance of a glucometer as a thermometer showing me when/if I am not behaving/looking after myself. I still take medication for it, but only one tablet daily rather than the four I used to take.

I want to share with you that anyone can get depression with a severe medical diagnosis, but when we see it as a wake-up call, it opens our eyes and invites us to change aspects of our life for the better.

Bonnie Hoo

Chapter 43

DEPRESSION - How I Took My Power Back

Mental Health is something that I am really passionate about. In the past, I remember being on prescription drugs for depression, attending counselling sessions and using other self-help services but not really getting anywhere with it as a teen. It was so frustrating and I had no clue what to do.

Lucky for us, we now live in a time where we have modern technology; so, me being me, started researching online for answers. I even started looking into self-development because I knew that I could be a better version of myself and it would definitely help me on my journey to healing because I had lost so much confidence and self-esteem. I got myself a mentor that was already successful in the areas that I wanted to change, which if I must add was the most expensive thing I have EVER invested in BUT was the best investment I have made so far. It taught me to invest in myself. It helped me to be more accountable and responsible in my life. It stopped me from making excuses for why I can't succeed in life and encouraged me to think bigger and step out of my comfort zone, which helped build my confidence more. While building a lot more meaningful relationships, not only with myself but others around me too.

On my journey, I experienced being a service provider as a mental health support assistant, for those struggling within my local community, through a group, one to one. The support, plus giving away free mental health self-help books, gave me faith that supporting others by offering these services were helping decrease suicide rates. It was this same self-help book that started my journey to recovery. It helped me realise that I should never stop learning, I won't always know the answer and do I need to know the answer? if I wanted change, it starts with me taking steps to change, it taught me that I am the creator of my own reality and I thought it would be a great way to give back by sharing some of my story.

Late October 2020 was hard. A close friend needed me and due to the choices made, he sadly grew his wings. It really broke me. I thought that was me completely finished, back to square one. I had an interview on the local radio about our campaign we had running the day after I found out. I do not cry often but I cried and cried. I felt like I failed him. I knew he wouldn't want to see me the way I was, so I had a word with myself, pulled myself together and did the interview.

I realised I could do more, so I wrote a mindset hack handbook. In the handbook it teaches you more about cognitive behaviour patterns, how they affect our lives and how to find solutions to those problems that we face on a day to day basis. I am working on many more projects, building an army of people to help turn things around, a group of like-minded people that have been on a tough journey but have seen the light and want to help others. I have learnt so much over the last few months, from being more aware of myself and others around me to being more present and expecting less and that's where I learnt the most, on how to take my power back.

When I decided to train to become a Cognitive Behavioural Therapy (CBT) practitioner at the beginning of the pandemic, I didn't really know what I was getting myself into. Halfway through the training, that's when it hit home. It really hit me hard at first. I thought the trainer was savage. How rude. Is he allowed to say that!? The words echoed in my head, "Go check yourself, you are stuck in victim mindset! You are not a victim at all but you choose to be because you want to be the victim. Full of excuses and quick to blame everyone else but yourself".

After a few days of it finally started sinking in, my teacher had given me the biggest wake-up call ever! I then started testing some of the techniques, I used the breathing exercises, taking deep breaths in for seven seconds, hold for four seconds and release for three seconds. I began looking at the relationships that I have with myself and those around me, asking myself regularly questions such as, am I being toxic in any way towards myself and others? Are the people in my life toxic? Could there be anything I could do to better my relationships? I started making time to observe and then respond, instead of feeling the need to respond or react before thinking and analysing the situation etc.

I started looking at potential outcomes and concentrating on the most positive outcomes, I started writing daily affirmations, breaking my day down into ten minutes sections, focusing my energy on something more fun and productive but also spending more time out of my head and into my heart.

Surprisingly, it worked. I am not asking you to believe me, try it yourself and you will see. I was sceptical at first but after trying the technique a few times, I noticed results. I feel more confident, focused, calm, more in control of my life and thoughts, the way I respond to outside influences and my attitude towards life has changed, that's just to name a few.

I started to make it a habit to do hourly check-ins with myself, I'd stand in the mirror and be honest with myself, I acted as though I was supporting a friend. Asking myself questions such as, "How are you feeling? What can you do today that will take you that step closer to your goals? Who do I need to build a more meaningful relationship with today? What toxic habits or people do I need to let go of today? What can I do today to reach my highest potential? What is my why? And why? I learnt that it is all about being self-aware, being able to observe and respond well in relationships, not only with other people but with yourself.

After almost fifteen years of battling with depression, it was those simple lifestyle changes that we are often advised to make, such as eating healthily, exercising regularly, drinking plenty, looking at your environment to see if has positive influences, reducing stress levels, being productive and having FUN. The help from other people also helped me throughout my recovery.

You know those sayings such as good food equals good mood, exercising daily (mentally and physically), goal setting and believing in oneself. As much as most of us would like to achieve such actions alone, the truth is that no one ever succeeded alone. As I said at the start of the article, we are so lucky to have the technology we have nowadays, all the information is out there. You can search keywords such as "mental health tips" or "how to look after your mental health" but one of the things that helped me the most was getting myself a mentor or coach. Someone that has been through the same or something similar and has managed to maintain a healthy mental health state.

There are many free courses and paid courses but if you really want to get better, you will have to invest time, money and energy in doing so and it won't happen overnight. On average it takes around sixty-six days to make a new habit automatic. So, if you start today, you may see some results within two to three months. It seems so farfetched. Well, they help and they help a lot. The more I got to learn about the brain, human behaviour and oneself, the more things got better for me. I attracted more like-minded people, more opportunities appeared, toxic habits, environments and people disappeared from my life and my health physically and mentally got better.

If you are serious about taking your power back or helping others to do the same, you can find the details below for my coaching and mentoring programs, free self-help books, CBT sessions and more by contacting me using the information below.

Are you ready to take your power back and start creating the life that you want?

Samantha Nicole

Neurological

"Health is much more
dependent on our habits
and nutrition than on
medicine"

John Lubbock

Chapter 44

I Believed I Could Heal ALS

I, Mr Kim Cherry, was sixty-three years old when I was diagnosed with ALS (Amyotrophic Lateral Sclerosis) on November 22, 2011. This was after some sixteen months of tests and misdiagnoses, leading to open-heart surgery and unproductive treatments for asthma, emphysema, and Chronic Obstructive Pulmonary Disease (COPD). My condition was advanced and I was told that my ALS was fatal, unstoppable, and untreatable. I was told that the normal survival time for PALS (Persons with ALS) is three to five years from diagnosis. In a visit with my primary care physician just a few days later, I was told I had a year, and that I would never see two. I was diagnosed with both Lower Motor Neuron and Upper Motor Neuron, or Bulbar ALS.

I am a successful businessman, entrepreneur, engineer, and inventor. To hear such declarations from doctors that I had come to trust was disheartening at best, and contrary to my whole life's approach to obstacles. After a few days of serious contemplation from the original diagnosis, my wife (Kay) and I made the decision that we would not accept the prognosis and that we would do all in our power to fight this disease. The doctors discouraged us from seeking any alternative therapies, saying they would only take our money and give us false hope. Though they said there was nothing more they could do did not mean there was nothing we could do. False hope is better than no hope.

I refused the only FDA approved drug for ALS, Riluzole/Rilutek and the "opportunity" to attend an ALS clinic. I felt the ALS clinics are there to measure decline, offer the next prop to the grave and give you no hope to heal.

By mid-January 2012, we decided to end our association with everyone, friend or professional, that was not positive and did not believe we could beat this disease. The power of the mind is a huge part of healing any disease. My traditional doctors refused to see any benefit from or initial holistic steps.

In early December 2011 shortly after receiving the diagnosis, we went to a Chiropractor, Dr Jared Nielsen, in Heber City, Utah, about three hundred miles from our Idaho home. He did some testing and said I had mercury poisoning, fungus, and gluten sensitivity. There went the homemade bread. I started the supplements he recommended to help with glutathione production and fungus reduction.

Faith in God, special religious blessings, and the love and prayers of friends and family, as well as our own prayers, have played a huge part in my success. I believe God helps those who work to help themselves. Through our internet research which Kay heads and still continues today, and tips from family and friends, we found things that have worked for us.

I recognize that this insidious disease is different for most everyone that falls under its curse. The primary challenges I faced were my ability to breath, and my ability to swallow, both Bulbar issues. I simply could not get enough oxygen and felt I was slowly suffocating most of the time, but especially at night when lying down, sometimes taking twenty to thirty minutes to work my way down from a propped up sitting position. I was choking on liquids, and even on my own saliva. My lungs were filling with fluid. My hands and forearms were rapidly declining, my right calf had atrophied considerably, and I had lost most of the strength in my right leg. I had severe drop foot, and my ankles would turn at the slightest misstep. Though I could still walk, my balance was shot. I was losing my ability to speak. I felt I simply could not get enough air to make the words come out. Walking more than a couple dozen steps required a breather, and a simple flight of stairs was daunting, requiring a mid-climb rest and a couple minutes recovery at the top. Also, the cold air seemed to almost shut my breathing functions down. I was experiencing severe muscle cramps, especially in my feet, calves, and thighs, sometimes experiencing two or three cramps at the same time.

We started with Dr Nielsen's program immediately. Things did not get immediately better. About the middle of January, I survived a couple of the worst nights of my life, sitting up all night on a sofa, fighting for every breath. It was then that I started using supplemental oxygen, which really helped.

By late January, we started seeing improvement in my ability to breathe, though fatigue and strength were still serious issues, as was the cold. But perhaps one of the biggest benefits of meeting with Dr Nielsen is that he was the first professional that told me I had a good chance to beat the disease. Not only did I believe him, but I believed that he believed it too.

In April of 2012, we added ozone and hyperbaric oxygen treatments to our protocol. The treatments with the ozone and hyperbaric therapy originally took from four to six hours a day. I gave myself intravenous (IV) ozone three times a week for the first two months, then cut back to two times a week through most of 2012. I had an IV port placed in the summer of 2013, which greatly simplified these treatments.

I mentioned earlier that my improvement has been phenomenal. I started playing golf again, riding a cart, in March of 2012. We sold our primary business in June 2012.

We spent the winter of 2012-2013 seeking warm weather and lower elevation to help with my breathing issues. When we returned from Texas in the spring of 2013, I knew that I had made great progress.

In the summer of 2013, I had my mercury fillings replaced by biologically safe methods. Also, in the summer of 2013, we decided we could not just stand by and let others suffer if what we had learned was helpful, so Kay began a website and continues adding to it monthly. You may reach us through it, should you like to contact us.

I continued to have hand and leg cramps periodically, up until November or December of 2012, but now seldom have any, even after walking a round of golf, as long as I make sure I stay well hydrated. I was also able to start swimming again. Staying hydrated at the beginning was difficult as fluid was going into my lungs with every swallow. Drinking carbonated water stimulated throat muscles to help with that problem. In three years, my throat muscles completely healed.

The supplements we felt were the most important are magnesium for muscle issues, alpha-lipoic acid for toxins and free radicals, lion's mane mushroom to rebuild myelin sheath around the nerves, astaxanthin for free radical damage and oxidative stress, turmeric with black pepper for inflammation, CoQ10, Vitamin D3, Vitamin B12. We also used Essential Oils to help heal the spine and Breathe Essential Oil to help my breathing. Using a magnesium rub or magnesium lotion can help those occasional muscle cramps.

Food changes included going gluten-free, eliminating sugars, and changing the oils we used. Coconut oil is the best for PALS. We eat mostly organic foods and meats grown without antibiotics and hormones. We got rid of cleaning chemicals in the home and found "clean" sources. We changed the personal care products which are loaded with bad chemicals. We suggest PALS get rid of soda pop, alcohol, tobacco, and other unhealthy products including all fast foods. I had become and continue to be very sensitive to tobacco smoke, perfumes, colognes, and other similar products as they shut my lungs down. However, the smells of the natural essential oils never bothered me.

My progress on my reversal continued slowly for the first six years, but I had a major setback in early 2018, due to an infection of my IV port. This resulted in two hospital stays, the first for two weeks in February and the second for ten weeks mid-May through July, a battle with sepsis, two mini-strokes and a second open-heart surgery. The biggest carry-over from this setback is constant vertigo, which has greatly affected my golf game and ended my swimming and bike riding. Though I still have some ALS symptoms, particularly with my gait and balance, and of late with my breathing, I expect to continue to heal. I may never be completely free of the disease, but I can LIVE with what I have.

Best wishes and God's speed to all PALS.

Mr Kim N. Cherry

ALS survivor

Chapter 45

My Healing MS Journey

Fifteen years ago, I was severely suffering from Multiple Sclerosis (MS) symptoms. I was sick. I felt like a stranger in my own body and it was terrifying. It started when I suddenly lost vision in my right eye.

Following a visit to the Emergency Room (ER), there were a plethora of tests; MRI, blood work, spinal tap, physical exam and a four-night stay with intravenous steroids and fluid all while wearing a patch over my right eye. (At this point I was more traumatized by the spinal tap and loss of vision than the thought of this maybe being a chronic autoimmune disease.)

After my hospital stay, I was diagnosed with Multiple Sclerosis at the age of twenty-four. The twelve months that followed are quite a blur. I was completely exhausted. It was the kind of exhaustion that leaves you with no control of keeping your head up or your eyes open. My whole body was tingling, I had muscle spasms in my neck and shoulders, restless legs that kept me up throughout the night, shivers, chills, massive anxiety attacks that crippled my speech and movement. I had brain fog and couldn't remember a thought and some days I couldn't remember certain words. I was so depressed and lethargic that at times, I didn't know why I was still alive. All I thought about was how much pain and suffering I was feeling. I found no joy in life.

To manage my symptoms, I took a disease modifying medication known as an interferon which I had to self-inject every day. I was also taking a handful of pills for muscle spasms and tension, anxiety, depression, acid reflux and asthma. After a year of living with MS and managing my symptoms with pharmaceuticals, I had this nagging thought that would not leave me. It was a voice in my head that was saying "the medicine is making you sick". All I knew was that I felt worse on all this medication than before I was diagnosed, yet this medication was supposed to be helping me manage my symptoms and stay healthy. Healthy was something that was so far away from my thoughts back then. I just wanted to not feel terrible.

At this point I was taking a multitude of pharmaceuticals. After consulting with my neurologist, it was clear that he was not supportive of my idea of stopping the medications and he expressed fears of a relapse. I don't know what it was that came over me, but the idea of getting off of this medication left me with more hope than fear and I can't explain why that was, but I clung to that glimmer of hope.

Then, I began the journey of weaning myself off my pharmaceutical medication. My husband and I took to Google and through our own research online found out that most MS symptoms are caused by inflammation. I then researched natural ways to reduce inflammation. This was in the year 2006 and at that time there was little information online about the impact a healthy lifestyle had on managing chronic illness and autoimmune disease.

This was the beginning of my healing journey. I did not set out to heal the MS. I just wanted to manage my symptoms naturally and holistically without any pharmaceuticals. Over the next few months, I did the best I could with the information I found online and I radically changed my diet. On a side note, I would like to say that what I did at the beginning of my journey is not what ultimately worked best for me in the long run and my needs changed as I got older and changed my living and working environments. When I first began my radical lifestyle change, I ate organic non-GMO whole foods. I did not eat any fast food, food from a can or overly processed food. I stopped drinking alcohol. I stopped eating dairy, red meat, gluten, and sugar. I added superfoods, anti-inflammatory foods and drank green juice every day.

As I changed my diet, my pain reduced quickly and drastically. I had less muscle spasms, less nerve pain, less brain fog, less anxiety, no panic attacks, and I began to feel connected to my body again. I started to feel in control of my body movements and in control of my thoughts.

As my pain lessened, I had more energy and began to think clearer and feel more hopeful about the future I began to practice changing my mindset. Now, at the time, I did not know that was what I was doing, I just knew that I did not want to have negative thoughts any longer. These thoughts were stubborn since I was consistently thinking them every day for the past twelve months. I began a practice of positive affirmations and gratitude journaling every day. As soon as I woke up, I would think about three things I was grateful for in my life. I would take to my journal and write these things down. I would look in the bathroom mirror and say positive affirmations like, "I am healthy, I am strong, I am capable, I am loved, I am safe". And throughout the day, when I had a negative thought like "I am so exhausted", I would quickly say my positive affirmations, smile and shake it off. Literally, shake it off. I started to move my body in order to reconnect with it. I started practicing yoga and I would stretch throughout the day. Massage and movement were so important to re-establish a connection with my body.

I found more ways to have fun in my life and find the joy that I had lost. I would dance, color, jump on a trampoline, write, walk outside, play on a playground, and play with my food! Anything that made me feel alive.

I revisited my neurologist some six years after I had decided to live holistically, and my first MRI after being drug-free for six years had improved. My lesions had healed. That seemed miraculous but then another six months later, again, my lesions healed. My neurologist stated that if he would have seen this most recent MRI on day one in the emergency room then he would not have had enough to diagnose me with Multiple Sclerosis. I was validated. I am healing. This is possible. I am listening to my body, I am speaking kindly to myself and moving through the world with the intention to feel connected to my body, mind, and spirit. I was told to just keep doing what I was doing.

Now, fifteen years after my diagnosis, I am happier and healthier than ever before. I am symptom-free and when people ask me what the secret is to beating MS, I say that it is to focus on Food, Movement and Mindset. But ultimately, everyone is different and will be affected differently. In my professional life, after my diagnoses, I followed my dreams. First, I worked as a paralegal, next for a non-profit as a crisis intervention advocate for women who are victims and survivors of domestic violence and sexual assault. I then became a restaurateur, created and opened up a local farm to table restaurant that had a juice bar, seasonal menu, and served beautiful organic food.

All of my professional paths were extremely fulfilling but now I have found my true calling as a certified holistic health coach. I created a health coaching practice that allows me to work with women who have Multiple Sclerosis. I help to navigate holistic options to overcome chronic fatigue, anxiety, and debilitating symptoms in order to get back to living a life of love filled with more energy, balance, and joy. Through my journey living and healing MS, I have learned how to listen to my body, live life fully and passionately, learned how to identify what my needs are and how to satisfy those needs, how to love and adore myself and how to connect authentically with my community. I would so love to connect with you and thank you for listening to my story.

Patricia Dickert-Nieves

Chapter 46

Healing Starts with You; Five Steps to Self-Healing

I have been on my healing journey for many years, after I was diagnosed with Amyotrophic Lateral Sclerosis (ALS) aka Lou Gehrig's disease and Motor Neurone Disease (UK), in 2002. Even before going to a neurologist for a diagnosis, I was working with many alternative and energy healing practitioners; almost twenty years, learning how to work with energy and doing energy healing myself.

I used many different techniques, each one teaching me something different. There was no one thing that healed all the issues I had, so I created my own practice for healing that works for me and I stopped the progression of the illness many years ago, using a combination of energy healing, dietary, environmental and mindset changes. I want to share what I've learned so that you can create a practice that works for you.

I discovered Dr Bruce Lipton and his book, The Biology of Belief, early in my healing journey and this quote became the cornerstone of my healing strategy;

"It is also important to note to fully experience your vitality it takes more than just getting rid of life's stressors. In a growth-protection continuum, eliminating the stressors only puts you at the neutral point in the range. To fully thrive, we must not only eliminate the stressors but also actively seek joyful, loving, fulfilling lives that stimulate growth processes."

I believe that the body knows how to heal and it's up to us to support it, to remove stressors and bring in love and joy. We support our healing and health with a positive mindset; removing obstacles to healing like stress, limiting beliefs and toxins; and increasing energy both internally and externally. This strategy can be done with traditional and alternative treatments.

Five Steps to Self-Healing

1 - Achieve and Maintain a Positive Mindset

2 - Emotional Energy Healing

3 - Detoxify Chemicals and Heavy Metals

4 - Increase energy from Internal Sources

5 - Increase energy from External Sources

Step 1 - Achieve and Maintain a Positive Mindset

The first step to achieve and maintain a positive mindset was for me to know and that I could heal. I never gave up and kept exploring. I searched for and connect with people who have or are healing, who inspired or motivated me. What did these people do? How did they do it?

After being given a (terminal) diagnosis of ALS, instead of worrying about what might happen, I continued living as if I wasn't going to die...

Even while doctors were trying to figure out what was wrong, I was working with an incredibly supportive group of alternative and energy healing practitioners and I kept trying treatments, supplements and energy healing. I kept the ones that helped, discarded the ones that didn't and continued to try new ones. I NEVER GAVE UP.

Where possible, I limited the amount of time I spent with negative people. Unfortunately, I couldn't avoid all the negative people and messages, but I learnt to limit the impact they have on me and my attitude. I chose to FOCUS on the positive messages, not on the naysayers and negative ones. I generally ignored people who had a limited view of what's possible.

Focus and Visualization

I chose to powerfully focus on health, abundance and love. When you look at yourself as whole and perfect, things may change to reflect what you focus on. I spent more time every day imagining myself doing the things that brought me joy and I felt the joy and freedom, as if I was doing them. When you change the way you look at things, the things you look at change, through your focus. Whatever it is, choose it and focus on it, powerfully focus. Knowing that healing is possible is critical to healing.

Step 2 - Emotional Energy Healing

For me, the second step of my self-healing, emotional energy healing, has been very transformational. I am not the person that I was before. I was so unaware of what I was experiencing in my life. Due to insecurities and self-worth issues, I did everything that I could to distract and numb myself, rather than feel the feelings. I was in a constant state of stress for decades.

When I say emotional energy healing, I mean a method that clears or releases trauma, and stress triggers, so that you remain in a healing state. Some of the methods of emotional energy healing are Healing Codes, Emotion Code, Quantum Energy Transformation, Emotional Freedom Technique (EFT), The Wonder Method, and more. There are many techniques that are simple to use and you can learn from a book, audio program or you can hire a practitioner.

Keeping a journal of issues to clear or release, including but not limited to issues and people that caused my stress; past trauma; limiting beliefs to what is possible; limiting beliefs to loving myself unconditionally helped too.

Now when I feel something, I feel it, acknowledge it, love it and allow it to leave. I have spent years doing the inner work clearing trapped emotions. I learned emotional and physical self-care from doing inner work and I feel better about myself now than I ever have. I learned that I am lovable, I am worthy, and I deserve good things. I don't need anyone to give me love and approval, I can give it to myself any time that I choose.

Step 3 - Detoxify Chemicals and Heavy Metals

I detoxified my body by changing my diet to organic, non-GMO foods and using natural personal care and household cleaning products. I also eliminated toxins from my body using an infrared sauna and supplements.

I use lots of products from vibesup.com and other earthing products, to protect me from Electric and Magnetic Fields (EMF) and cell phone radiation.

Step 4 - Increase energy from Internal Sources

Even when my mindset is on track and I am in a healing, rather than a stress state, I need energy to repair. I increased the level of healing energy in my body through meditation, which also reduced stress, increased energy flow and energetic frequency.

At times, I simply sat quietly while feeling love and joy with a focused breath. I used Quantum-Touch, which has the same benefits as meditation, for healing as it works through breath work and focused intention on love.

I also used Qi Gong, Tai Chi and Kundalini Yoga because they are well known to increase energy and have healing benefits.

Step 5 - Increase energy from External Sources

Even when my mindset was on track and I was in a healing state, I needed energy to repair. I went outside and sat in the sun, with my bare feet on the ground. When I couldn't get outside, I used Earthing.com and VibesUp.com because they bring earth energy indoors. Other devices bring light indoors, bright light, Red and Near Infrared.

Being indoors around electronics and EMFs is stressful and inhibits healing, so since I spent a lot of time indoors, I have many tools to energize me like; light therapy, crystals, essential oils and structured water. I have been "structuring "my water for many years. I have devices that use vortexing and sacred geometry. I also filter it and use crystals and other energy healing tools.

The Daily Practice

This includes both inner and external work to eliminate toxins, increase energy from nature and use healing tools. We are all different, so our practices will be different.

A couple times a day, or as needed, read or listen to inspiring messages.

Review your Journal and add any new issues, check in to see which ones need attention and do some healing.

Meditate or do Quantum-Touch remembering to give yourself Love, Approval and Gratitude.

Go outside to be in nature, use energy devices, drink structured water, use essential oils.

Avoid toxins in your food, water and personal care products.

Dawn McCrea

Chapter 47

With God's Help, Healing Myself Following a Stroke

I had been under some unbelievable personal stresses – but like so many – I PUSHED THROUGH THEM, and ignored the signs of what was to come.

My fiancé, Sandra and I, were out in the parking lot of a bookkeeper that we had used – and she was going to 'run in' and speak with the owner while I stayed in the car, as we still needed to make it to the office. Out of the blue, I couldn't move my right side, I thought it was my imagination. It got worse over the next five minutes, so I decided to call my fiancé inside the bookkeeper to alert her. It was then that I discovered that I struggled to speak... "OMGoodness", was this going to be 'it' for me? I left a garbled message at 09:38 on her phone – and by the time she got back to the car (10:00 AM), I had no capability of speech or right-sided movement. Atypical yes – but when it happens to you – it's very real.

Ambulance was called. Paramedics grabbed me and hustled me into the ambulance and took me to the premier stroke facility in the area. Once I arrived, they had come to the same conclusion, and since I was within the three-hour window, gave me intravenous drugs to dissolve the clot. A scan however showed a rather large section involved in my brain, so they proceeded to take me to the Operating Room to thread a catheter (tube) up my groin to the brain and again make another attempt at dissolving the clot. It was a "hail Mary" for sure, but emergent times call for emergency measures.

Immediately, Sandra had many people praying. The nursing staff told her to expect the worst and that I'd be in rehabilitation for the next three to six months most likely. I'd never practice as a Physician again. I wouldn't make it to the actual WEDDING we had planned for July 23, 2008, in Hawaii.

They hauled me off to Surgery and I didn't know if I'd ever make it out. I couldn't speak, I couldn't move and I was terrified of the prison my body had become. My brain (thought process) worked fine, and I communicated 'goodbye' and 'I love you' via blinking of my eyes to Sandra.

I awakened, groggy. My right hand DID work. I struggled but could speak a bit. It was a miracle. But my miracle still had a lot of work necessary going forward. I was let out of the Intensive Care Unit after three days, and sent home with a prescription for Coumadin/Warfarin (blood thinners), which I refused, and orders for a Physical Therapy evaluation. I refused to go as an inpatient to a facility. Stubborn like I am, I knew that I could do more on the OUTSIDE than if I was there.

Immediately Sandra had taken me to my office, and, at my instruction placed me in my Hyperbaric Oxygen Chamber at 1.5 ATA pressure. I had done this for other patients, and I prayed that it would work for me too. Studies in 2005 showed that Hyperbaric Oxygen Therapy (HBOT) increases our healing stem cells as well as helps with developing new blood vessels to supply injured areas.

I accomplished forty hours of HBOT in two weeks, and my body had indeed responded! My movement became more fluid. My speech was ungarbled. God had spared me, and I was recovering. I cannot stand to be immobile, and I insisted on being in my office (with a light schedule) and saw patients in the office.

PURPOSE helped me to heal. I had refused the Coumadin/Warfarin, as I had seen it cause too many problems for others, and had begun taking WOBENZYME, a natural agent that helps prevent and dissolve clots. I was determined to make it.

I made it to our wedding on the Beach in Maui on July 23, 2008. That in itself was a miracle.

I continued my own rehabilitation when I returned to the mainland, and began another round of HBOT. I performed the scalp Acupuncture on myself, as nobody seemed to know about it! I used Microcurrent stimulation for my muscles, was strictly clean with my diet, and PRAYED nonstop. God delivered me from the worst.

Miraculous as all of that is/was, I had more miracles in store. I had been a Hockey Player and was determined to at least begin SKATING once again. I was strong enough by September 2008, and laced up the skates for the first time. Difficult, but it worked.

I did reflex activation and hand/foot/eye coordination drills every waking moment, including video games as soon as I would get out of the Hyperbaric Oxygen Chamber. Beginning these drills after maximum Oxygen input to the Brain – i.e., turning on the vulnerable areas of the injury, where HYPERBARIC helps re-set the brain's response after injury. This the PEAK TIME TO TEACH THE BRAIN! I did ball/hand juggling and bouncing drills, and would do the same with my feet on the floor, controlling a ball with each Hyperbaric treatment. I would even bring a soft rubber ball INTO the Hyperbaric Oxygen Therapy Tank to see what I could learn. I used every waking moment that I didn't have something else occupying my time.

By the end of September 2008, I put on my hockey goalie equipment and went to an 'open' scrimmage to test the waters. God's miracle was continuing to evolve, and I was BACK BABY!

I began the Hockey Season in October with a team that did not know what had happened to me. I didn't want them to take it easy and I also wanted NO PITY. God had gifted me with recovery. I played. In a very short time, I played WELL. By Christmas, I was completely 'back' as far as hockey was concerned. The guys on the team could not believe that I had indeed had a stroke. I couldn't either.

The Neurologists were dumbfounded. I wasn't taking their prescriptions. I wasn't doing the LAME physical therapy that they wanted to put me back into! They asked me to be in an observational study (which I did for a year) to monitor my progress. When I would discuss the benefits of Hyperbaric Oxygen Therapy, I was 'dismissed', but they could not argue with the outcome. They said I was 'lucky'. BULLCRAP. I was healed and BLESSED BY GOD, and my therapy worked.

Since that time, I have added many additional techniques that have enabled me to assist my patients with the same affliction, including augmenting their treatment with Stem Cells as well as Cold Laser Trans-Cranial Therapy.

As always, the most therapeutic effort I ask all patients to spend time in prayer and visualize their own healing, and to help direct the body where to concentrate their healing reserves.

Alexander Thermos, DC, DO

Chapter 48

Healing from Brain Injury

How it all started.

In March 2013, I fell off my horse. It started with a headache. A few days working from home, I thought, and I'll be fine. But every day it became more difficult. The strain of working, even of doing daily tasks like cooking, became more difficult, leaving me drained of energy and in such pain. Still, I tried to push through it, surely it would improve soon if I kept trying?

Five days after the accident, I opened an excel spreadsheet full of formulas I had created myself. I couldn't understand any of them. Had I really created this document?? Not some mathematical nerd? I was scared. Had I become stupid? Would I ever have the same level of comprehension and logic that I used to have?

On day six, again I woke up with a heavy head. A dull, thumping and foggy feeling, like I wasn't really there. Dazzled I looked at myself in the mirror. Two dull, brown eyes were staring back at me. I burst into tears and asked myself "why?" "What is happening?"

I had sustained a brain injury but I had no idea what that meant. My life had stopped and I was no longer able to take part in society. But still, I was alive. This was the first moment that I realised there is a life outside society. These days I would say: if you fall out of society, you fall into life.

No help was offered by any doctor or hospital and the common advice was to do as much as I could to try to participate in society. There was an expectation that you have to accept your situation for the rest of your life. But I wanted to heal. To me, it feels so unnatural not to want to search for ways to heal, so I chose to follow my own path and do all I could to heal myself.

My path of self-healing

Energy work

After the accident, reading was almost impossible, I didn't understand the words on the pages, it was just dazzling and I couldn't remember a single thing. I spent time every day, trying to read and understand a few lines in a book, simply to give me the idea that I was actually doing something. Computers were even worse because of the flickering of the screen.

In a magazine, I discovered an article about energy healing, using your own hands. Even though I couldn't read, mimicking the images looked simple enough. I followed the pictures and gently started embracing each finger. Immediately, my whole body started to react. I alternately felt warm and cold sensations. I started to yawn and burp. I felt a little sick, my muscles were quivering, my head buzzing and my body was tingling. In the end, I fell asleep.

The morning after I was taken by surprise; I clearly felt better than I had done over the past weeks! From that moment on, I treated myself daily with the energy techniques of Jin Shin Yiutsu. After this, I learnt reflexology, Reiki and other healing methods and techniques, including AuraChakra healing, Heart Coherence and Feldenkrais.

Even though working with energy is a great support, it doesn't bring a spontaneous recovery. During the first year, I treated myself for six hours a day on average. By doing so, I developed a deep body awareness.

In addition, I underwent treatment from various energy-based therapies, including Cranio-Sacral Therapy, Shiatsu, Touch of Matrix and Eye Movement Desensitization and Reprocessing (EMDR). The energy work truly energised me and rebalanced my brainwaves. It helped me to recover from the strain of my brain being overloaded, allowing me to be more active.

As well as the energy work, I physically trained my brain through the doing of activities, stimulating my brain cells without overloading them, to regain those activities and functions in my life. I have learnt to understand the language of my body on a very subtle level and discover the best ways to regain functioning.

Meditation

All day long my mind was buzzing with thoughts about all and nothing, not in the least with worries and fear. But quickly I came to see that constant thinking was a burden to my brain. I decided that my mind had to become quiet. This was easier said than done, but after a few weeks of meditating I succeeded; for a fraction of a second there was nothing. What a feeling! Now that I have found the place of silence, I have succeeded in getting there more often and for longer periods. Now, some days, I don't have any thought for hours during the day.

The effect of meditation on my brains was stunning. The pain reduced and the brain fog became less dense. During the day I slept less because meditation gave a deeper rest than sleep did.

A very in-depth process followed in which I discovered how meditation could literally bring about healing.

Self-reflection to heal

I realised that my life up to this moment had led to my current situation. If I wanted to get out of it, I had to change. Healing doesn't happen from outside and can't be arranged by others. You have to do it yourself from the inside out.

Looking in the mirror, what my inner self presented me with was painful. I was willing to see, but that didn't make the process of transformation any easier. Feeling, digging, crying and gaining new insights followed. Acting upon them, making different choices and changing my behaviour; changing myself. Self-reflection became a life attitude. Convictions, beliefs, thought patterns, were they all true? What were my habits and what was their foundation? How did I feel and why? Nothing escaped my attention anymore and I kept peeling off layer after layer, to the core of me.

Creating a new life

Many of the insights I gained are bundled into my Dutch book 'Eigentijdse Wijsheden'. After such a long period of little functioning, it felt amazing to be able to do something as special as creating a book. It was published on October 3rd, 2014.

I wanted to use my experience to inspire others, as life had inspired me and I started teaching mediation and coaching people in their healing process. I wrote a new book in support of achieving a better recovery from a brain injury that was published on October 3rd, 2017.

Brain injury a second time

In 2018 I sustained another brain injury from a car accident. Once again, my life stood still. I saw one advantage; I now knew the way. However, the first question was why did it happen? What life lessons did I have to learn?

By getting deeply in touch with my intuition, I gained new insights. It showed me that there was more personal transformation to be done. I was invited to discover my true self on a still deeper level. I was invited to discover my own voice. I was invited to step into my power, to let my inner light shine more. I was challenged to find the strength to stand for what I believe in and to act accordingly, to no longer hold back and make myself small. By transforming my perceptions and attitudes, I resolved once again what had been limiting me to feel free to be myself.

Health is no longer something I take for granted. I work every day to maintain and further improve it. I enjoy it. It's normal to take care of your body and do self-work. It is fun to change your worldview and free yourself, taking control of your life, discovering and making use of your talents, creating a new you.

Key sentence

The image you hold of yourself, the world and life, translates into health and is the key to healing

Stephanie "Joyous Mind"

Author of

Eigentijdse Wijsheden

Chapter 49

MS Stands for "My Story". You Write the Pages of Your Life, Not the Illness

was diagnosed with Multiple Sclerosis (MS) at the age of twenty-two when I literally just woke up sick one day. By the age of twenty-five, I was in a wheelchair. This wasn't the life I wanted to have.

The doctor prescribed me medications that left me shivering on the floor, in the middle of summer, as if I had malaria. At one point during my treatment, I was given an intravenous (IV) drug that had a side effect of causing Progressive Multifocal Leukoencephalopathy (PML), which damages the brain, literally brain rot. I was terrified.

This was around the time Facebook was evolving and through it, I saw all my friends from school graduating and having families. I was sick with MS and felt as if my future was bleak and my life was going nowhere.

MS can change day by day as well as hour by hour and affects everyone differently. One day I would be walking around and then suddenly find myself collapsed on the ground; no balance, no coordination, no short-term memory. The memory issue associated with MS caused me problems at college where previously I'd had a GPA of 4.0, but in just one semester it dropped to a 2.8.

I felt so negative with it all and really struggled with my mental health. At the time, I couldn't focus on anything good because I was taking medication that made it worse. Every day, I was sick and it was a constant battle, like struggling with the flu. It was hard to be positive.

At the time, I weighed one hundred and fifteen pounds and was so skinny. Some days I could walk, and other days I kept collapsing and had to be carried out of my job. Life at that time was a rollercoaster. I went to the doctor, with my little brother to assist me, to see what medication to try next. My brother saw the doctor search the internet to find which medication would help me. That really opened my eyes because if he could do that, I could too.

As we left the doctor's office that day, I felt a change in me. I decided I could help myself to heal and I was going to do it my way. When I got home, I threw all the medication in the bin. Yet, the doctor had warned me that if I stop any of my medication, the MS would get worse and I would go downhill much quicker. I just wanted a few more years of not being sick every day. I was sick of being sick.

I was introduced to a book called *The Secret* by a friend who is a nurse. This book talks about the energy of positive thinking and the law of attraction - that the energy you put out is the energy you get back. When I first read the book, I thought it was a pile of crock, how can being positive affect life that much.

At this point, I was willing to try anything and thought, what have I got to lose?

I started making myself small and achievable goals. It wasn't that long before I started noticing that I was achieving these, plus more. That's when I realized there was something in it. I focused on staying positive, no matter what. It was a slow process but I was doing it.

Then I started researching which foods would help with healing. I learnt about healing illness the natural way, through diet. Prior to MS, my diet was poor. Like every college kid, I was eating junk foods. So, I made changes to my eating, taking a more natural approach, choosing foods like bananas and chicken. I radically cleaned up my diet. That was a huge step in the right direction.

I decided to start exercising and went to the gym. I had never been to a gym before. On my first visit, I sat peddling slowly on the stationary bike and watched other people work out. I noticed that the more I bicycled, the less pain I had in my legs. It felt energizing, so I decided to go to the gym every day. As I increased the resistance, I had longer times without pain in my legs. I knew this was the right thing to do in my healing and I wanted that feeling more and more.

As my weight increased, it became an instant addiction. People started noticing and complimenting me on my physique and I loved the changes in my body. These changes pushed me forwards to do more. I kept going and going.

MS for me was the greatest thing that ever happened. As crazy as it sounds, it radically changed my life, so I am thankful that I got sick. My MRI in 2010 lit up like a Christmas tree, showing the MS but a repeat MRI in 2017, showed no active signs of it.

Everything that I went through was a struggle but I now feel like there was a reason for it. I use my experience to help others who have been diagnosed with MS, all over the world. The first thing they tell me is their MS diagnosis. I try to get them to understand that they are not their diagnosis. The diagnosis can be a setback, but a setback can also be a step up.

As we change our thinking to accept this, it can lead to something great in life. I understand that it's hard to get out of that mindset, but there is another way. I did it, I went against my doctor's advice. It's not easy, but you just gotta try. You have to find a way, there is always a way and the path is never set. I never allowed myself to focus on failure.

Most people think once you're in a wheelchair, you're stuck in a chair. You're not stuck with MS. Most people think MS is the endgame, but it's pretty much changing every minute. If you're going downhill, change course. Changing your life and trying to be healthier is not going to hurt you.

These days, I have a good job, an amazing wife who supports me and a little daughter. Life is great.

My Transformation Tips

1. Shift How You Think

You have to reprogram how you think and start believing that you can do things or at the very least, try to do things. It can be hard at the start, but over time it becomes a mindset.

2. Take Control of Your Own Health

You can't let the diagnosis of a disease be who you are. I threw out my medications because they were making me sick and I started studying nutrition and changing the way I thought. I took control of my own health. Find something that you are passionate about, then focus on the passion rather than the diagnosis.

3. Never Focus on Negatives

A bad day is not a bad life, it is just a lesson learned. Don't think of it as a setback. You may fail a few times, but it's not going to hurt you as long as you're changing your life by trying to be healthier and more positive.

4. Use Setbacks as a Step Up

When I was diagnosed with MS, I was in a relationship and we broke up. This motivated me to change. Find a way to use setbacks as motivation rather than discouragement and turn them into steppingstones.

5. The Only Failure Is Not Trying

I was already in a wheelchair and feeling sick every day, so what did I have to lose by trying something new? For me, making the decision to give exercise a try turned out to be the best decision I ever made, for my health and to reverse the MS.

What are you waiting for?

Kevin Smith

Chapter 50

MS Left Her Totally Paralyzed; Homeopathy and Lifestyle Changes Reversed It

I t was our son's thirty-second birthday and I dreaded calling him and his brother. I had just taken their mother to the Emergency Room (ER) for the first time in their life. We thought it was nothing serious. The day before, she felt tingling down her right side. That morning she woke up slurring her words and had poor balance. Doctors suggested that it was probably a stroke and began stroke medication immediately.

Daily hospital visits revealed her condition worsening. The swiftness, violence, and rapid deterioration of her condition confused doctors. On the fifth day, she nearly died. CODE BLUE! Every doctor and nurse on the floor rushed to save her. She couldn't swallow, so they intubated her and added a feeding tube, before sending her back to the ER.

A perfectly normal, working, walking, and talking woman was, within five days, totally paralyzed. She could not speak, walk, talk, swallow, or control the movement of her eyes. There was no prior medical history, personal or family, of anything like this.

The doctors were stumped. After they had given dangerously high amounts of steroids and intravenous infusions of immunoglobulins, they said that they had no more pharmaceutical medications available to them that could abort or reverse this process. It was at that point that I vowed to give her Homeopathic remedies as I knew they could do no harm and would assist recovery.

She was transported to a second hospital for seven days of Plasmapheresis treatment. A spinal tap and multiple MRIs revealed lesions in the brain and spinal cervical region, confirming a diagnosis of Relapsing-Remitting Multiple Sclerosis (RRMS).

Doctors told us to prepare for long-term hospital care and, probably, a wheelchair for life. They suggested Multiple Sclerosis (MS) drugs to prevent future relapses. Doctors also recommended cancer drugs because the immune system was attacking itself. She said NO to both types of drugs and began taking daily natural Homeopathic remedies.

What did my wife do to Reverse MS by ninety-five percent?

My wife has always had the "mindset" that our thoughts, attitudes, and emotions create our health condition. Our physical body is a reflection of the mind. Now, she had the challenge of putting her knowledge into action.

While in the ER, within the first three days, and while she could talk, I began asking my wife questions. We knew that if she could identify what caused the issue -- stop the stress -- she could reverse this drastic health condition. What caused this worsening health condition, paralysis, and stress? How did this condition serve her and what was she trying to learn?

She was working in a new city, a new job, trying to get a permanent position, and back home our house was being renovated. We were preparing to sell, so we could move closer to her new work office. Lots and lots of stressful decisions.

She had reached a point of maximum stress and the physical body reflected that stress with MS. She realized in the ER that her thoughts of stress, anxiety, and fears had brought her to this point. She accepted it and began fixing it straight away. She began to release her stress and fears and relax her physical body. Many times a day, she repeatedly built up her visualization and intention of her body fixing all the issues.

After eight weeks in the hospital, she was transferred for a fourth time to a rehabilitation hospital, as doctors suspected that her positive attitude might make her a good candidate to benefit from intense physiotherapy. She regained the ability to swallow food and water safely.

At this point, she could not get out of bed or transfer to a wheelchair by herself. She had to be moved using a mechanical hoist. She made great progress relearning to use her upper arms, hands, and fingers including moving her head, but her core strength was low and her legs were still too weak to hold her balance.

At the rehab hospital, she finally gained enough strength to transfer from bed to wheelchair and walker. This was then followed by hours of physio, occupational therapy, and more self-imposed exercising at the gym. Every night during sleep, she would play YouTube videos of Louise L. Hay to help her sleep and to help her reprogram her mind.

She meditated, practised relaxation, visualization and positive affirmations, every day. She had an extremely positive attitude and wore T-shirts at the hospital with positive messages on them. She chose not to focus on diet as she was eating hospital food for four months. Later, she also added pool therapy, balance exercises, and Chiropractic treatment.

She refused to say or accept the MS diagnosis and refers to it merely as an event in her life. After four months she walked eighteen meters and out of the hospital, for good. Today she can walk more than fifteen thousand steps a day (9+ km) and she has returned to full-time work.

She has learned to express her feelings and as soon as stress starts to build up, she releases it by expressing it and relaxing, both physically and mentally. We sold our house and moved closer to her job so that she can walk more and get more sunshine. She changed everything about herself, including her lifestyle.

MS is classed as an autoimmune disease with no known cure. She was able to reverse it within two years without using medication. In the first two weeks, two doctors told her that she was unlucky with everything that happened to her. Now, they tell her that she is so lucky to get better so quickly.

She feels that everything she did combined to synergistically help her reverse the condition. She felt in complete control of her healing. On the last MRI, it is clear that her lesions are disappearing. Three years later, she continues her regiment of Homeopathic remedies and Louise L Hay visualization exercises to promote a thriving lifestyle.

For more info on using natural remedies to reverse MS and other neurological conditions, please contact me through my website.

Domenic Stanghini

Other

"He who has health has hope; and he who has hope, has everything."

Arabian proverb

Chapter 51

Healing Depression and Fibromyalgia Through Release

Pain has been a constant presence in my life. As has disbelief in said pain. This made it really hard to talk about, I kept it to myself as I knew it wasn't "normal". I felt disconnected from friends and family, and most importantly myself. I became more and more depressed as I got older. In 2006 I was diagnosed with insomnia, anxiety and depression. All the while, the pain in my back and legs got worse and spread throughout my entire body.

In 2014, I was finally diagnosed with fibromyalgia, hypermobility and hypersensitivity. It took eight months of testing to get this diagnosis, I believed that finally knowing what the cause of all my pain and symptoms was would be the road to recovery, I was sadly disappointed. Being told I had this incurable, chronic disease that would only worsen over time was the worst thing I had ever heard. Needless to say, this increased my depressive state. I was anxious about doing anything for fear I would have a flare-up and was depressed about my life in general. I was self-pitying, angry and felt like there was no reason to keep on living.

I was working in London. The busy lifestyle and stressful work environment added further strains to my already weakened body and I eventually left my job and moved back in with my parents. Whilst living in London, I had begun to write poetry as a way to let out my feelings and frustrations. I was surprised at how cathartic this was and at first, I didn't share my creations. However, my mum read my work and loved it. I doubted that I was any good, even when other people said so. I kept on writing though and found myself making up poetry all the time.

I became more depressed as I was not doing a job I loved and I missed my friends so much but felt like I would be bothering them if I reached out. My mum took me to her botanical illustrations class and I really enjoyed it. I began learning botanical illustrations for myself. I found it would get almost meditative to be looking at a flower and drawing it and I would lose myself in it just like the poetry.

I was always an avid knitter and found this was a great distraction from my pain and the negative thoughts. I would knit gifts for my friends so they knew I was always thinking of them. When they told me how much they liked them it filled me with so much joy and I felt I was achieving something great, rather than just sitting around and feeling sorry for myself. I still had days when I wouldn't do anything creative and I found I was much more depressed, anxious and felt the pain more deeply on these days.

After the first lockdown began, I sought out a counsellor to help me. I felt surprisingly comfortable with her during our first session. It felt like I was priming myself to be open to healing. I started to use my DoTerra essential oils and crystals much more and looked for yoga videos that were more suited to my abilities, without feeling like I was weak or disabled.

My searches led me to Sarah Harvey and her meditation programme with The Self Healers' Society. During this, I felt more comfortable sharing things that I had kept to myself for a long time, such as my struggles, my fears and my poems. This was a very eye-opening, mind-expanding journey, I learnt so much. I journaled for the first time and let my creativity soar!! I meditated more, read books and watched videos on healing. I began tai-chi again and most importantly started to love myself and my body.

Believing that I can heal all the symptoms I have had for so many years was a pivotal step in the right direction. Every time someone told me that we can heal, I would refuse to believe it would happen for me. I found myself getting very defensive and telling myself tales of why I couldn't.

I had already started Cognitive Behavioural Therapy (CBT) for Depression Caused By Perfectionism. This radically changed my way of seeing things. Previously, I would strive for perfection in even the little

231

things in life and get so stressed and belittle myself when things were not perfect. Once I allowed myself to change this belief as well as many others, I began to feel happier and less stressed.

I have just been informed by my CBT therapist that I am no longer clinically depressed AND I would no longer be diagnosed as having a mental health condition now. This brought me to tears, it has been a long struggle, one that I never talked about because I was ashamed. Within six months of having CBT, as well as all the other forms of therapeutic healing I undertook, I healed clinical depression. The secret is to allow yourself to talk about it, write about it, meditate and journal on it. If your mind is keeping you locked inside of your own personal hell, how can your mind be the one to free you without any external help?

During this time of radical change and healing, I found my purpose. I have always wanted to help people which is why I became a scientist. But I realised I wanted to help people like me. I wanted to help people with chronic and mental health conditions to open themselves up for healing. I created Inspire Calm to coach people in how creative hobbies can facilitate healing chronic conditions.

I believe nurturing your creativity is very healing in and of itself. The pride in the things I have drawn, knitted, made or written really elevates my mood and replaces the negative, self-destructive thoughts. By changing what you are focusing on you can really reduce symptoms, even during a flare-up, which is when it is hardest to want to do something positive and creative.

I was always told to keep my hands busy, something I learnt from my mother and grandmother, they both taught me so many creative things. I realised how much joy these hobbies brought me and how much they helped in my healing journey. Now I find them to become meditative acts of self-love.

Tripat Riyait

Chapter 52

From A Bottle A Day to Nothing, My Battle with Alcoholism

My Name Is Raymond and I'm an Alcoholic.

Well, I know that now but I didn't know that when I was growing up in Ireland and always felt different. This is a before during and after ongoing recovery from alcoholism, which is a mental, physical and spiritual disease.

I was always a nervous kid. I always felt different from everybody else and was very shy. I found it difficult to socialise, meeting new people or strange relatives from across the water, so much so my own mother used to call me an oddball, something that didn't really fill me full of confidence going out to play with my mates. Hi, I'm Raymond the oddball.

When I went to work in an office, I found it even harder. I always hated people talking to me and I could feel myself going red in the face, almost to the point of crying. Other people would pick up on this which exasperated the whole situation.

My older brother and sister used to drink quite a lot and I didn't like the negative changes I would see in their personality.

While working in the office job a colleague introduced me to alcohol at lunchtime, a bottle of Harp lager which I didn't like the taste of until he put a dash of lime in it, then it slipped down easily. Later in social situations, I found this helped me socialise and lose my self-consciousness. It also helped me lose my Civil Service job as I use to fall asleep at my desk after lunchtime sessions. I was just about eighteen at this stage.

I moved to London and did various jobs but at twenty-three, when my mother died, I noticed an immediate dependency on alcohol. You see with her death, I immediately developed panic attacks and my cure-all, alcohol, took over my life for a good eight more years. I went very quickly downhill both mentally and physically. I also became dependant on sleeping tablets which I used ironically to cut my drinking.

In the meantime, I met my wife, got a job in a club as I couldn't afford my addiction and quickly was on my way to rock bottom. On leaving the club each evening, I would put an empty litre bottle to the vodka optic, put in my ten shots of vodka, top this up with tonic, six cans of lager and even put a load of ice in the bag. I was then happy as I had my nightcap.

My father passed away while I sat with him and my older sister in the hospital. Before he passed, I had a conversation with my sister, asking how she had managed to stop drinking. I was sitting with a quarter of a bottle of brandy in my inside pocket, just in case. It was always "just in case", just in case I had a situation I couldn't handle.

My sister had told me about an organisation called Alcoholics Anonymous (AA) which she attended. I couldn't work out how a group of people sitting in a room talking could rid me of this addiction. I believed that nobody drank like me.

I attempted to go to a meeting but when I peeped inside the window all I could see were a lot of chairs in a circle facing each other. I couldn't handle this because of my self-centredness, so left and continued to drink for a further two years.

Eventually, I picked up the phone to AA. They got a member to contact me and take me to my first meeting on St Patrick's day. I thought what is an Irish man doing in an AA meeting on St Patrick's day. However, I was amazed to hear a man who was ten years sober share a drinking story very similar to mine. From that day I knew I was in the right place and not alone.

I began going to meetings on a regular basis but five months into it I picked up a drink and went on a drinking session that lasted five days. I was very quickly back to square one and I knew what I had to do. I got back to meetings and worked the twelve-step program and got a sponsor (mentor).

Later, during my recovery, I helped others while still on my own road to recovery, you keep it by giving it away. My liver is normal, my appetite is more than normal and I find it easier to communicate with people. I gave up sleeping tablets shortly after giving up alcohol. I did this in a controlled way and did not use any form of mood-altering medication to come off alcohol and I still don't use any medication today.

They say when you pick up a drink you stop growing emotionally and when you put it down after many years of drinking, you go back to the emotional age you were when you picked it up.

Well, that's my story of recovery cut down in size. I am not representing AA, all I can say is, it was the only way for me to give up my addictions. Often people seek medical help and get referred to rehabilitation centres, which can be very effective. From there, they are introduced to AA.

For me, it is working this twelve-step program a day at a time that keeps me sober, no medications, no drugs and most importantly no alcohol.

I found the twelve-step program to be a spiritual program. I was told the difference between religious people and spiritual people is that religious people are afraid to go to hell but spiritual people have already experienced their own hell.

In the twelve-step program, I admitted I had a problem, found a higher power to hand things over to, looked back on my past and shared it with others. I cleaned my mind, made amends to those I had hurt, worked on my defects of character, made new amends when necessary and passed the message on to those still suffering from alcoholism.

I went on to get a great career and was able to retire early and enjoy my sobriety each day. I practice meditation and work on my spiritual program in my own way. However, I know if I don't do this my way it works better for me. When I thought I was in control and followed my own advice, listening to a voice telling me to drink and it will all be ok, it all went wrong.

On September 11th 2019 I was 30 years sober.

Raymond Patrick

Chapter 53

Healing My Inner Self to Heal My Symptoms

I always knew deep inside of me that illnesses do not happen out of the blue, rather they are a signal from the body telling us something is not right. I remember that I used to have skin rashes on my face as a child when things were going badly in our home between my parents. I grew up in a household of domestic violence, so life was full of fear. I have come to learn that skin problems can arise from fear and anxiety. After my parent's divorce, my skin cleared up.

I also remember that I had shingles at the end of my final year in high school. I believed this was because I was highly stressed and did not know what I was going to do after my graduation. I was desperate and under pressure. Once I worked out a plan, the shingles healed. I understand that Shingles can develop from fear and tension.

During my sabbatical with a friend, through the Caribbean, I had ringworm on my left leg. It totally makes sense to me now because my friend "got under my skin" with her constant aggression and looking for trouble. I have always tried to avoid conflict. I never really learned how to resolve it or set boundaries. I now understand many years later that the reason why I felt so irritated and chose to cut contact with her was that she reminded me of my childhood, when I was at mercy of someone or something.

During my career in corporate fashion, I use to suffer from gastrointestinal problems all the time. The doctor's examination had proved that there was no physiological or dietary explanation. I know now that it was a way my body telling me that I needed to make a change. I was very unhappy with what I was doing, thriving for a career in a big corporation I thought was my personal choice. I was depleted, depressed but was too afraid to make a change to something completely different so I kept on going. I thought my solution was changing companies or positions but it wasn't. I remained unhappy and in pain.

Only when I took a leap of faith in 2012 and quit my whole life at that time: job, apartment, city and country, did the pain go away. I knew I had to make these big changes otherwise I would have ended in burnout. I planned a six-month trip through the Caribbean. All I wanted to do was to go surfing, practice yoga, explore, and be at ease with life, without any further plans and leave everything behind. I know now that my gastrointestinal symptoms represented my biggest fear; fear of new things, of change and the incapacity to digest something new at that time.

My six-month trip turned into five years, in the Caribbean. On the one hand, I was living life more in flow and doing more of the things I genuinely enjoyed. I was much happier and without physical pain. On the other hand, I was still carrying depression with me every day, numbing the pain with parties and alcohol. I did not understand why I felt empty inside of me. I never felt true happiness within relationships, so couldn't have a healthy relationship.

During my journey abroad I truly got to know myself better, through a lot of introspection. I met all my demons, unresolved childhood trauma through people such as that old friend, relationships etc. I went through the dark night of the soul, right there in paradise. I felt like the loneliest person on earth. I tried everything I could that promised healing, from chanting mantras, reading books, astrology, getting more familiar with spirituality, distant healing sessions, I tried anything I could. It did help me to feel better and have social contact, which I had avoided for some time. However, the depression I was in was not healed. The relationship I was in was unhappy, I had no desires and my periods stopped.

Hurricane Irma destroyed the entire island of Anguilla where we were living at that time, in 2017, so I returned to my hometown Köln in Germany. The place I left at the age of twenty and never thought I wanted to return to. I was lost, without a plan and homeless. I moved back in with my mother. The same house where I spent my childhood.

However, it worked well because I was able to improve my relationship with her.

I was determined to take my own healing into my hands. I wanted to resolve the depression, my absent periods and now, I was diagnosed with an underactive thyroid. I refused the pharmaceutical treatments that my doctors wanted to prescribe and they warned me of detrimental health consequences for not taking the drugs. That is when I came across the teachings of Louise Hay, Dr Joe Dispenza and others, who confirmed the ability of self-healing.

I signed up for coaching programs which helped me understand my childhood traumas fully and I was finally able to release all the remaining stuck emotions which I had stored inside of me for many years. Additionally, with the help of my yoga practice, pranayama, meditation I was able to re-connect to my feelings. I'd learnt to disconnect from them as a child, to survive the pain of domestic abuse. I also learnt an understanding of spiritual realities and with tremendous self-work, I finally felt depression free for the first time in my life. Depression is known to be caused by unreleased emotions!

I've learnt to actively speak my truth and express what I am feeling and thinking, unlike before where I held everything back because I learned that speaking out was unsafe and therefore meant fighting. I also used visualizations and affirmations telling myself and getting into the feeling that my thyroid was in perfect health. Learning to speak out, feel and affirm has all helped me heal.

With regards to my absent periods, I consulted a wonderful homeopathic practitioner specialized in phytotherapy. She recommended a buckwheat fasting for ten days, in addition to an individualized tea for my condition. At the same time, I finally realised that my relationship was not going anywhere and that I was not living my truth by continuously planning my life with this man. I was clinging on to a person and a life that were no longer mine. "The day" I separated from this seven year relationship, my period returned.

I am living proof that self-healing is possible. That is why I made it my mission to guide others in their self-healing journeys. I re-invented myself as a transformational coach applying holistic coaching tools and yoga therapy to guide "depleted high achievers in overcoming physical and emotional challenges so they can make a shift into a life aligned with their hearts desire". They are my former "I".

My self-healing journey rewarded me with abundance in all important areas of my life. Now I am ready to help guide others in their healing process.

Angie Kim

Transformational Coach & Yoga Therapist

Chapter 54

Rock Bottom Health Due to Vitamin D Deficiency

2014 was the year I started asking questions. Why was my health rock bottom! I seriously had, had enough of feeling like I was, constantly ill. Nothing I did ever seemed to work. You see as a child we were encouraged to eat mints if we had a cough, and take medication for a cold! All my life I had chest infections one after another and every year they seem to get worse than the last one.

This last chest infection went on for months in 2014 and I was losing all my energy to fighting it. It was as if it was here to stay for the rest of my life. Yes, I'd had enough of it. It was getting to the point where it was so painful, I couldn't breathe. I always had a tight chest and felt low all the time. I believed that I would never get better. Little did I know back then that it was reversible.

This is where I started asking questions and started on my healing journey. I had this passionate drive within me to get to the root of all my illnesses so that I could prevent further chest infections for the rest of my life. What drove me to find healing was my daughter. We had sixteen years' worth of labels, diagnoses and many medications. Nothing brought a cure but they all created new ailments and everything affected her body and mine.

I didn't know at the time but there are no cures for us, only preventatives. I wrote all her ailments down and started connecting the dots. The more I looked at it, the more it became clear to me that the body works as a whole.

I found solid evidence that led me to understand my health or lack of it. Something simple!

I continued researching and asking questions in different support groups. The more I dug into my ailments, the more I understood, I had a VITAMIN D DEFICIENCY. The symptoms fitted neatly into the bigger picture that I was building.

I referred myself to a rheumatologist through my doctor and asked for a vitamin D blood test to see what my levels were. (That simple!) My rheumatologist confirmed that I did indeed have vitamin D deficiency, as well as hypermobility, Sjogren's syndrome and linked to Ehlers-Danlos syndrome. All autoimmune system problems and caused by the amount of inflammation.

I declined the strong tablets that I was being encouraged to take, as I didn't believe medication really worked, after watching my daughter suffer. I started to believe it was all due to vitamin D deficiency and I had passed this on to my daughter through my genes. I could see at this point how all my ailments could be prevented, through the supplementation of vitamin D3.

I was given a prescription of 10,000 International Units (IU's) of vitamin D3. As I started taking it, I knew it had raised my levels because my cough and chest infection were disappearing and it was helping to clear all the inflammation from my body. It was such a relief to feel well. I also knew within those first few weeks that I would be on it for the rest of my life.

After several weeks of supplements, my rheumatologist advised me to drop the dosage down from 10,000 IUs to 2,000 IUs. I did as I was asked because I thought my rheumatologist was right. Boy was I wrong there because within two weeks all my ailments started coming back.

At this point, I knew I couldn't rely on our National Health Service so I started doing more research and taking responsibility for how I was feeling. It's no one else job to make me healthy except for me. I joined a Facebook site for vitamin D deficiency and started learning more. I soon realised that I needed to increase my dosage.

After increasing my dosage to 5,000 IUs, I started listening to my body and learned to spot the signs of ailments returning. This was because my body was getting used to the amount of vitamin d3 that I was taking, so I felt I had to increase it every so often.

I also realised that I had to take other vitamins (co-factors) with vitamin D3 as it depletes the body's stores of magnesium. I started supplementing magnesium, as well as vitamin B12, K2 and omega3. My weight had increased to thirteen stone at this time. My joints become weak and I was unbalanced and I felt the constant weight of my whole body.

I was introduced to natural, plant-based phytonutrient dense products by friends. I changed my diet and did shakes of fruit, vegetables and berry capsules. After four months, I was seeing incredible results. I was slowly losing some of my excess weight. I was fighting inflammation and replenishing my cells, I had more energy and better health. I was firing that flame within me and healing. My cravings stopped and my ailments reduced as I stopped eating all the wrong foods and overeating.

Five years on and my health is still improving. I'm growing and learning more every day and my mind is so much clearer than it has ever been. I have lost three and a half stone and I feel happier within myself. I am constantly maintaining my health and wellbeing and building on my daily routine to achieve what I have.

I have changed what I listen to and turned off the television because it is so negative. My body picked up all the low vibrations from all this negativity. I read more books and now fill my mind with good knowledge. I learn from people like Tony Robbins and I now have a Tony Robbins trainer in my life whom I'm very friendly with. I know when I need help and guidance, he's there for me.

Yes, my beliefs were holding me back and I'm now learning to breakthrough them too. I'm learning about meditation and how that works for me too. I have positivity and affirmations in my life now. My diet is the best it has ever been, although there is still a little room for improvement in places. I am walking so much better than I used to do and can now walk eight to ten miles a day.

So, you can see just how I've become a better person wholeheartedly and I have now become one with myself. It hasn't been easy. I never gave up building up my vitamin D levels until I was pain-free and today, I'm taking 80,000 IUs of vitamin D with all the co-factors because it helps connect the whole of my body together.

My journey carries on and I just keep on keeping on. I now have happy, stronger tissues than I had five years ago.

My Life is a journey and it's a beautiful one as my challenges become my victories and to have health that is one hundred percent better than I had, is just one victory.

Heidi Foster

Chapter 55

Healing Epilepsy and Osteoporosis Without Pharma, Against Medical Advice

Following a traumatic custody battle between my parents, custody was given to my mother. Everything seemed to be going well until my periods started at thirteen years old and I started with grand mal epileptic seizures, for which I was prescribed anticonvulsant drugs. The seizures left me feeling like I'd ran ten marathons as well as not really being in touch with the world, for around ten days after. I totally lost touch with who I was, as the medication made me so drowsy.

My seizures happened after being woken quickly from a deep sleep, never when I was awake, and always during my periods. When I spoke to the specialists at the hospital, explaining that the seizures only happened during my periods and the medication was making them worse, I wasn't believed and they increased my dose, causing me to become zombie-like, negatively affecting my school grades and my energetic, bubbly personality.

After being on it for eight months and it making me so drowsy, I found myself slumped in the doorway of a shop. I was not going back to school; I was angry and frustrated. I found myself wandering around in a second-hand bookshop and picked up a book, for just 25p, written in 1968, about alternative healing.

It documented that those that suffer from any form of epilepsy, have deficiencies of calcium, magnesium, manganese, selenium, zinc, vitamin A, vitamin B6 and B12, vitamin D, and taurine. Activity was recommended; walking and swimming, and having baths with

Chamomile and Lavender, the use of essential oils, changes in diet included adding essential fatty acids and Vitamin E, eating plenty of vegetables and proteins, drinking infusions of Chamomile, while avoiding pasta, bread, sugar.

The following morning when Mum put the tablet on my tongue, I stuck it on the roof of my mouth so when I stuck my tongue out, it looked as though I had swallowed it. I went straight upstairs to the bathroom and spat it in the bin. I did this every day.

I then withdrew all the cash from my bank account, bought everything listed in that book and began my secret natural healing journey! I was inhaling the orange, geranium and ylang-ylang essential oils from the bottle and fell in love with feeling in control of my body. I had my first aromatherapy soak in the bath with my Chamomile and Lavender and this was the beginning of a lifelong happy relationship!

In just over a week, I would be due my monthly period. I was calm and feeling the benefits of the natural supplements, the essential oils and feeling really switched on, not at all drowsy. My period came, was not as painful and heavy as my usual bleed, no flinching, no twitching, sleeping soundly, waking up slowly. I was feeling wonderful and in control. My next visit to the hospital for an electroencephalogram (EEG), six months after being on my natural treatments, showed a marked improvement. I was THRILLED to announce my natural therapy discovery!

Moving forward to age thirty-two, I was enjoying work, and had fallen in love with my best mate. Life was finally coming together until I read an article in a magazine that the contraceptive injection I was having, was linked to a decrease in bone density. I had been on it for over seven years and the maximum time for this prescription was one and a half years. I had a bone density scan and the results were not good at all. The doctors warned this could be bone cancer.

My Grandparents had always said, "even in the darkest heaviest clouds you will always see a silver lining". Whilst awaiting the results of the tests, I did some real deep thinking. Talking with my sweetheart I told him that if the tests come back negative, I want to quit my job, sell my apartment, sell everything, buy a bus and tour Europe. It was the most scariest, yet thrilling moment of my life, WE AGREED!

Thankfully, my results came back alright, although I had the bone density of an eighty-year-old woman. The doctors wanted me to take an alendronate drug for life, advised me to drink more milk, not drink coffee and stop my high impact gym classes. WHAT? I had an active life of aerobics, salsa dancing and going to the gym. Still, my sweetheart was thrilled I was Ok and we continued with our plans! We handed in our notice at work, put the apartment on the market and began selling everything.

I began the once-a-week medication which burnt my throat and the effects on my body felt like flu; I felt heavy, painful and sore. I returned to the Doctors and explained what I felt when taking this tablet. Unmoved, she told me they were for life. I remember being told this about my epilepsy medications and the lightbulb went on.

I began researching. My search led me to a wonderful holistic practitioner who after my first email responded with "I will help you, I want to help you". With that, I dumped my tablets in the bin. That evening, my sweetheart returned home with a book on osteoporosis which explained that should you have this bone disease your system will be leeching calcium, you have to learn HOW to absorb calcium, a yin and yang theory. When you eat dairy you also need to eat nuts, when you eat fish you need to also eat vegetables, it was fascinating and all about balance.

It explained there was more calcium in broccoli than milk. It listed recommended supplements of Vitamin C, B, D and E, Calcium, Magnesium, essential fatty acids and apple cider vinegar. Spirulina algae powder and nettle tea were also recommended. So, I increased my usual supplements and got my life back again. Aromatherapy was back in a new capacity!

It was during this time that I began to have really bad cramps from what I thought was perhaps stress. After tests, it was discovered that I was borderline celiac, so I couldn't eat gluten; pasta, bread, biscuits, pizza. I just wanted my new life!

Soon, the apartment and possessions were sold, we left our careers, bought an American Winnebago, said our goodbyes to England, headed off touring France, Andorra and Spain, to have the best time of our lives. We were on a course of healing our bodies and our minds, NATURALLY!

We settled at a campsite in Spain and loved it. After three years of continued natural supplementation and living the Spanish life, I underwent another bone density scan. I was now considered "low-level Osteopenia". OH WOW! CHAMPAGNE TIME! We went to our favourite local restaurant and my sweetheart had a pizza and I had my vegetarian dish. I tasted his pizza; it was divine and then I waited for my body to react to the gluten in it. No reaction.

The next day I tried a baguette, no cramps! We went to our local health food shop where we had been purchasing my supplements (a very emotional moment). I told them the good news of my bone density scan and that I had no reaction to the gluten. They explained that by my taking Spirulina algae powder, I had healed my gut. Imagine how happy I was!

I've since read about the "ALENDRONATE BLACK BOX WARNING", so many deaths linked to this prescription, AND there was no evidence that alendronate actually re-built bone! I am SO very grateful to have found a path that led me to all the natural healing that healed my symptoms and for my sweetheart who has been my strength throughout. Here I am now, minus seven prescriptions.

All these experiences have led me to train to be an aromatherapist and sell essential oils, which has given me the most magical of experiences! When carrying out client treatments, sometimes, I have been drawn to a certain area on their body where I find myself throwing away an unseen energy from that area. My clients hadn't even realised there was a problem, until it was gone. "How did you know?" they ask, my answer is, I don't know. Maybe it is the voice that pushed me into the bookshop? Maybe this is the voice that put the medications in the bin? whatever, I am TRULY grateful for THE most life-changing course of events, for without them I would never have thought I would ever be living in the Spanish mountains, with my sweetheart, my four much loved dogs, leading a completely different, a VERY HAPPY LIFE!

Vanessa Lewis

Chapter 56

Emotional Healing Led Me to Physical Healing

I n January 2020 I was diagnosed with Hashimoto's Thyroiditis, Endometriosis, Adenomyosis and a leaky gut. The Hashimoto's led to many symptoms such as mild headaches, heart palpitations and pain, high cortisol and high oestrogen, horrible gut issues like food sensitivities and bloating and very poor sleep. In regards to the endometriosis, for years I struggled with unbearably painful and heavy periods, low back pain, and swollen breasts before menstruating.

Healing has been a journey and it really started with focusing on my food. I already ate a very clean diet with a lot of fruits, veggies and pasture-raised, organic meats. After my diagnoses, I went on the Autoimmune protocol for eight months which was really restrictive but I felt amazing on it! In the beginning, I could only eat about seven vegetables due to food sensitivities which I found challenging. As time went on, I was able to add in more variety. I eventually transitioned off as I didn't want to develop any more nutrient deficiencies. Little did I know that food was not the thing that would heal me.

In regards to supplements, I went on a leaky gut protocol and put a lot of focus on liver support and detoxification. It took months for me to see a difference in my gut health, but I kept taking my supplements religiously, knowing it would eventually pay off.

I would say my healing journey really started in April 2020 when lockdowns started. I lost my job which allowed me to take the time to really slow down and get more in tune with myself. I started to open up spiritually which has been such a gift. Instead of heavy weightlifting, I focused on low-intensity exercises such as walking and yoga to bring my body into a parasympathetic state. I stopped forcing my body to exercise and started honoring how she felt. I started meditating and journaling daily. Allowing words to flow out of my pen with no judgement was a pretty paramount turning point for me. This is where I started to break down the emotional walls that I had put up.

Healing the physical body has everything to do with healing the emotional and spiritual body because they are all so deeply connected. Mind-Body-Soul. I had always heard the phrase but it never really struck a chord until I was at my lowest low with my health. One night as I laid in bed meditating and was in another dimension, I heard a voice saying "healing is within you". I immediately burst into tears and knew, although my gut was still completely wrecked, that I would one day heal. I wouldn't be stuck like this forever. The next day I saw a significant improvement in my bowel movement and bloating. It felt like a miracle, but that it was the power of my mind and probably my spirit guides sending energy healing. The beauty of it all is we can rewrite and rewire our brains for healing.

After that night, I started practicing the affirmation "I am healed" and really FELT what it would be like to be healed. I would have dance parties during my affirmations, which are still a daily occurrence, getting me into my feminine energy. We cannot heal if we are not in our feminine energy. It allows us to receive the healing that is our birth-right.

In October 2020, I started to feel stuck on my physical healing journey as I was falling back into old negative mindset habits and had stopped doing affirmations, daily meditation and journaling. I had gone back to work which gave me less time to do all the personal development exercises I was so used to doing every day. I was extremely ungrounded which caused a lot of anxiety and being irrational. This was another layer of healing I needed to focus on. When we are not grounded, we are disconnected from our body, our heart and our connection to Source. Getting grounded is very challenging for me as I am often up in the clouds and quite analytical. Making grounding a priority has allowed my racing thoughts about healing or life in general, to just float away. When I allow myself to get ungrounded, my physical body also suffers because I get stressed.

At this point in time is when I started getting into energy healing. Energy healing has been the real catalyst for my healing. It has allowed me to release and remove energetic blocks and work through emotions that have been stored in my body my entire life. Since we are all made up of energy, we simply cannot just focus on the physical body but must focus on the entire mind, body and soul as a whole. Without each one, the body cannot heal. And chronic illness is always caused by trauma and stored emotions.

After a specific energy healing session with my coach, my body temperature which was almost always at 96.6f, went up to 98.7f and has stayed there ever since. If you have a hypothyroid, then you can resonate with always being cold and having cold hands and feet.

During this session with my coach, I found out that I, myself, am a powerful energy healer. So, I started practicing on myself, which has been absolutely incredible. Having the power to heal yourself on so many levels is absolutely mind-blowing. At this point in time, I was running a Hashimoto's Healing Coaching business but felt very unaligned. Finding out I was a healer has led me into alignment with my souls' purpose; running my energy healing business. Being in alignment with life speeds up the process to which the body heals!

Another layer to healing was opening my heart up. My heart was so closed off that the energy from above was not able to move to my lower chakras and organs for healing. This is the reason why I have had such a stagnant liver, endometriosis and gut issues. Although opening my heart is an ongoing process, I feel amazing and am dedicated to growing and expanding every day. I have gratitude for the life that I have been gifted, struggles and all. Those struggles have made me who I am.

As I continue to shed the emotional layers and work through emotional blocks, I don't even worry about healing my physical body anymore. I know that complete healing is around the corner and is completely available to me as long as I continue to put in the work, healing my mind and soul.

Danielle Sims

Chapter 57

The Power of Healthy Eating Habits

W e live in a life period where more or less everything is focused on gaining fast results. We give up too easily if we don't see immediate results because we live in a state of rush.

Hay fever

For me, a raw food diet turned out to be one of the most powerful and healing ways of eating lifestyle. I prefer to say an eating lifestyle because we have to change our lifestyle in order to improve it. A raw food diet is based on 70% raw vegetables, 20% raw fruits and 10% nuts, seeds and cold-pressed oils, such as extra virgin olive oil. Fortunately for me, all this was very easy to find from the local farmers in Slovenia, in the Mediterranean area.

Before my raw food diet, I was suffering from hay fever. Sometimes it was extremely hard to work as my symptoms of hay fever were very disturbing. After a month on a raw food diet, all my symptoms of hay fever faded away. I started to add rice, potatoes, cooked vegetables and grains to my diet.

The most fascinating part of my raw food period was that during that time, I met many people that had also been on a raw food diet for years. Their experiences were far more fascinating. Some of them cured diabetes type two and high blood pressure. Diabetes type two and high blood pressure are consequences of poor lifestyle, unhealthy eating habits, stress and not enough of physical activity.

I also found and used the *Caremaxx Bionase*, which treats allergy and hay fever symptoms with light therapy, also known as phototherapy.

Reflux

It was suggested that my issue with reflux was a genetic disorder, as many of my relatives suffer with it.

During my pregnancies and after my second pregnancy, I had very painful stomach cramps, due to reflux. Sometimes, they lasted all night. I found that eating small portions of light food prevented reflux. I had several gastroscopies as my stomach cramps were very frequent and extremely painful. The results of these gastroscopies always diagnosed reflux and thankfully, no ulcers.

As soon as I stopped eating fried food and minimized the amount of processed food I was eating, the reflux symptoms disappeared. I had spent years blaming the stomach cramps on the amount of coffee I was drinking (four cups a day) until I found out that wasn't the case.

Since my diet and lifestyle is based mainly on eating vegetables and fruits with nuts and seeds, and only eggs as a source of animal products, I no longer suffer from reflux.

Low energy

Although many articles suggest eating breakfast, this doesn't work well for me. After eating breakfast my energy level decreases and I feel tired. The only thing I can consume until around mid-day is two cups of coffee with oat milk.

Coffee with oat milk provides me with enough energy until lunchtime, then I start eating foods with a low Glycaemic Index (GI), such as organic wholemeal rye bread with avocado and cherry tomatoes.

I have noticed that low GI foods make me more energetic and active without any feelings of hunger, while high GI food makes me feel tired and hungry faster. A low GI diet definitely helps to stay a normal and healthy weight.

I would never use products that are food substitutes as the powders tend not to be low GI. I prefer unprocessed fresh, food like seasonal vegetables and fruits.

We can't ignore the correlation between healthy eating habits and our health. We can invest in our future health by minimizing stress and maximizing the awareness of the importance of good eating habits.

Structured water

All water has different energetic signatures. Water stored in glass will absorb differently into our body than water stored in other containers.

I drank structured water from the glass bottle with a signature. I placed it in the sun to absorb the energy. The taste of the water was so different compared to tap water. I feel it helped energise me.

I wish I had more time to do further research, but I am in the middle of a career change and I need to do some exams to start working in social care.

Food and cancer

German New Medicine is definitely knowledge I should share to help people understand the implications of using food to prevent and treat cancer.
 http://www.newmedicine.ca/

Alex Korosec

Chapter 58

From HIV To Health

I t all started in 2002 when I was eighteen years old and I received the news of a positive HIV test. I felt my heart drop to the floor. I felt the life I knew was over, and that the healthy body that I had was doomed.

All my life I had seen in the media the images of people allegedly dying from AIDS. As a result, I thought I had received a death sentence. Following my diagnosis, I started to go to an HIV/AIDS doctor. She told me that I had to start taking medication right away, or else I would die soon.

At that moment, I asked what could I do with nutrition and exercise. But the answer was no, there was nothing I could do. Believing the doctor and feeling that I had no other option available, I accepted my fate and started to take the antiretrovirals.

It is important to realize that until I started to take this medication, I was healthy, full of energy, and didn't have symptoms of any disease. However, as soon as I started taking the medication, everything changed. Straightaway, I started to feel its side effects. I lost my energy, was always nauseated and bloated, and my hair started to fall out. From time to time, when taking a shower, I could not feel the water on my limbs.

At the same time, I started to lose muscle mass in my arms, while my rib cage increased by ten centimetres. Within a few months. I developed other body reactions; skin rashes, major muscle tears, and cramps

Mentally, I was feeling dull, depressed and couldn't get interested in anything. In fact, all this seemed very strange to me. I had no prior

255

symptoms of any disease, and suddenly, as soon I started to take the medication, I had a cascade of body reactions.

Still, I kept listening to others' opinions, fears and beliefs, and took the medication for twelve years straight. Although I felt my body declining and in pain, I was so brainwashed that I kept doing what society and the medical community said was the right thing to do.

However, in 2014, my intuition was getting keener. The little voice inside my head was getting clear and consistent, and I realized I had to pay close attention to it. For a whole month, every time I took the pills, I kept receiving the same message: "It's time to stop taking it".

Deep inside, I knew the medication was blocking my body from its natural ability to renew itself. In truth, I could also feel it and see it in my body. And now I know why. The truth is antiretrovirals are in fact chemotherapy, and I had been poisoning myself, every day for twelve years.

Meanwhile, during that month, all the things I had heard from the media and doctors were popping up in my mind. Yet, the peace and expansion I felt with the possibility of freeing myself from the medication was stronger. Rationally, it didn't make any sense, but my gut feeling was telling me otherwise.

After pondering and questioning myself a lot, I decided that it was time to take a leap of faith. After all, the message was so clear that I knew it was the right thing for me to do. Finally, I followed my intuition and stopped taking the medication. Back then, I believed I had a very dangerous disease. I believed that it was contagious and that I was somehow dangerous to other people.

After all, I believed I could contaminate someone else, and that possibility terrified me. I also believed that without the medication, the HIV could get out of control, I could get sick and eventually die from it. In fact, when I took the decision, the doctors told me that without the prescribed medication, I would die within a few months or a year at most.

But at the same time, I totally refused the idea I was going to die from AIDS. With this in mind, I believed I had to do something, and decided to take things into my own hands. As a consequence, I chose to take full responsibility for all areas of my life, and especially for my own health.

All things considered, I had to find a way to take care of myself. Nature as a source of wellbeing always made sense to me. As a result, I started to research for natural solutions to improve my health.

I began to watch summits, masterclasses, documentaries and to read about nutrition, superfoods, raw food and body detox. And most important, I also started to take action, applying my new knowledge to myself. By listening and respecting my body wisdom, I followed its messages and changed my diet. First, I quit sugar. Then dairy products, meat, fish, and lastly eggs. As a consequence, my gut kept getting better and better. No more bloating or constipation. The pain and the swelling were going away, I had more energy, and was feeling better day by day. As a result, this kept me motivated to continue my research and practice.

At this point, I had also learned about seeds, seaweeds, superfoods, mushrooms and all kind of herbs. I drank plenty of filtered water, tisanes (herbal infusions) and freshly squeezed orange juice. At the same time, I also removed gluten from my diet.

With my new diet, I was nourishing my body with high nutritional and easy to absorb foods, which allowed my body to detox from the medication and regenerate itself. Besides, I discovered essential oils, lymphatic massage, Ayurveda and fasting, which were also essential to reclaiming my health freedom.

Meanwhile, I also realized it was important to work on my mind and emotions. By this time, I was already meditating daily. I became more aware of the limiting beliefs I was holding, which were blocking me from achieving my goals. As a result, I understood it was also essential to release the emotional burden of past traumatic experiences.

After searching for a while, I found Emotional Freedom Techniques, (EFT), also known as Tapping. The first time I tried it, I instantly felt its power, and a new world of possibilities opened up for me. With EFT I felt it was safe to express my emotions, fears and concerns. I uncovered more limiting beliefs, I had no idea I was carrying with me.

With this intention, I was able to reprogram my brain, mind and energy.

I worked on my fears of getting sick and being rejected, on the guilt and shame I felt, and also on my beliefs about HIV/AIDS. The most valuable part of my whole journey, was to learn the importance of listening and following my intuition.

Intuition was the guiding force that took me from one discovery to another, helping me find my path. By using it, I discovered how to reclaim my health freedom by empowering myself. Choosing to follow my gut feeling was the best decision I ever made. I'm now free of any medication since 2014, and I didn't die the way I was told I would. In fact, many years have gone by, and I'm better than ever!

Actually, all I had to do, was to find the root cause of toxicity, eliminate it, and nourish my body and mind at all levels. It was an incredible journey, and today I am grateful for my life experience. In fact, not only has it allowed me to conquer my health freedom, but it also helped me find my life purpose: to help others achieve that same freedom.

In the end, I hope my story inspires you to also start your health ownership and freedom journey. To know more about me and what I do, I invite you to visit my website.

Thank you,

Joana Bonança

Chapter 59

Hyperemesis Gravidarum's Extinction

I was never more excited in my life than to see that positive pregnancy test. But like many women, my excitement turned to absolute horror as I soon found myself living day, and night on the floor in the bathroom.

Hyperemesis Gravidarum or HG was the culprit of my agony. They call it extreme morning sickness, I called it hell. Constant vomiting morning, noon and night. I soon realized I had lost 25 lbs in just a few weeks. I almost prayed for death to take me, but I knew I had to live for the baby's sake.

This was when I started to research. There had to be an end to this misery. Everywhere I looked the message was clear: nobody knows why this happens and it gets worse with every pregnancy! Not only did I want babies I wanted a lot of babies, but I could NOT go through an HG pregnancy ever again. I vowed to myself to find some answers.

I came across a blog from a woman who had eight children and she found that eating fermented foods helped her HG. Replenishing the gut with good bacteria was helping her! Some women talked about out of balance blood sugars being the culprit of HG. But I couldn't keep anything down and I could not attempt to eat sauerkraut. I continued to suffer until I was fifteen weeks pregnant, and suddenly it was over. The rest of my pregnancy and birth was a breeze.

I had a friend who kept talking on Facebook about supplements that balanced her hormones and probiotics that were helping people with gut issues. I contacted her soon started taking the probiotics, lots of them!

Three months later I found myself pregnant again. That positive test filled my heart with fear. If I got HG again this time, I had to take care of a seven-month-old baby on top of vomiting all the time. The future looked like a nightmare! I continued my probiotics faithfully and waited for morning sickness.

Some nausea came and I would eat some food and then wait for the vomiting but instead, I felt better. Food was actually making me feel good in this pregnancy. I never got HG again.

I have never stopped taking probiotics. Two more babies have joined our family since then.

Good probiotics and clean whole foods make healthy pregnancies and happy babies.

Bonnie Madrigal

Chapter 60

Reducing Blood Pressure with Intermittent Fasting

I was a post-war baby, born in 1951 when some foods were still rationed. My mother was ahead of her time and really into healthy eating. She worked full time and we were latch-key children, which was considered normal at that time. However, she always cooked from scratch and foods such as ice cream or crisps were very rare treats.

My mother raised us to consider medication as a last resort, using fresh food, water and exercise to heal, with occasionally, herbs or supplements. She also refused to allow me and my siblings to be vaccinated and warned anyone who would listen, of the dangers of using aluminium saucepans and cookware, as she believed then that aluminium caused Alzheimer's disease.

Because of her, I have the same strong belief that most illnesses and diseases can be cured without pharmaceuticals and am horrified that among most people of my age, there is almost a competition to see who is taking the highest number of medications, as if it is a badge of honour!

Throughout my life, I have rarely been ill, occasionally catching colds and only once catching flu. However, for as long as I can remember, my blood pressure was always high, usually 140/100. I was lucky enough to have understanding doctors, who just monitored me and didn't persuade me to take medication.

I kept my weight within the healthy range (although at the higher end of healthy!) and always exercised, so they tended to leave me alone, saying that I was a "worrier" and recommending that I do more things to relax, like yoga.

In 2006, I moved to Spain and after a few years, registered with the local doctor, who, luckily for me, speaks perfect English. Those of you who have Spanish doctors will know that they are thorough, love blood tests, and usually have a prescription for everything. On Saturday mornings at the local Pharmacia, you will see elderly people leaving with small carrier bags containing their medications for the month!

Three and a half years ago, during a particularly hot spell, I was feeling extremely lethargic, which is unlike me, I usually have plenty of energy, so I went to see my doctor. She sent me for blood tests and took my blood pressure. She was horrified at the reading and wrote me a prescription for beta-blockers, plus three other drugs to bring it down to a normal level. I explained that I didn't wish to take anything, but she said that at my age (then sixty-four years old), I was at major risk of a stroke, especially as my mother had had a stroke at the age of sixty-nine, and my maternal grandfather had had one at the age of fifty-three.

She frightened me somewhat, which was obviously her intention, so I did leave with my prescription and went home.

I finally accepted that I could not ignore my high blood pressure any longer and needed to do something to bring it down to a normal level, but without drugs. I was fit, going to the gym three times a week, playing padel once a week and attending yoga and Pilates classes. My weight was at the top end of the healthy BMI range, so I didn't think losing weight was the answer.

I decided to scour the internet for a solution (good old Doctor Google!) and I came across an article by Michael Mosley, who had developed the 5:2 diet (Intermittent Fasting), after trying fasting. His diet involves eating just five hundred or six hundred calories on two days a week. One of the changes as a result of the diet was the lowering of his previously high blood pressure.

I researched further and found that all types of intermittent fasting appeared to do this, and decided that, for myself, I would find it easier to do the 16:8 version, which means eating within an eight-hour window and fasting for sixteen hours. I rarely feel hungry when I wake and find I can usually leave it until one or two o'clock before I need to eat something, so decided to make my eating window usually between one o'clock and nine o'clock, although this would depend on whether I was home or not.

For me, this was easy to follow, as there is no restriction on what one should eat, or quantity, only when. The hardest part was when I went out with friends for brunch or breakfast, as they originally had a problem with me not eating when they were, but they are used to me now! I was okay because I did not feel hungry!

When out I do usually have a coffee (with sugar!), which is meant to be a no-no, but for me, it does not seem to make a difference. I also occasionally have breakfast, but only if I am really hungry, which is rare. I find that if I drink half a litre of water upon waking, and another half a litre before lunch, I am just not interested in food. The more you follow this way of eating, the less you feel hungry and strangely, you don't feel the need to overeat when you do eat

After about three months, my blood pressure stabilised at around 117/85 and has stayed around there ever since. I also lost around half a stone in weight, which was welcome, and found that if at any time, I want to lose more weight, I just have to cut out starchy foods from my evening meal, foods such as potatoes, bread, rice and pasta.

I can thoroughly recommend this method as a way of reducing high blood pressure, and also as a way of reducing weight.

Jill Law

Chapter 61

What Does It Take to Heal?

There are so many great healing modalities out there to choose from and just like me, you may have tried many of them.

I'm trained and certified in Aka Dua Level 3, Instant Miracle, Peace Process, High-Frequency Energy Healing, and I am a Reiki Practitioner.

Do these certifications really matter?

Well, I recovered from two major conditions that adversely affected my life before my training. Actually, before I even knew anything about holistic or energy healing. Often. I was asked how I healed and my response was "I made the decision to heal and refused to believe the doctors".

Let me share my story with Interstitial Cystitis (I.C.) or painful bladder syndrome!

When I was diagnosed with Interstitial Cystitis at twenty-four, I was in disbelief that I was dealing with this chronic illness at such a young age. I remember one day going to the doctor for the weekly treatment and thinking, I'm dealing with a painful chronic illness now, what am I going to look like when I'm sixty?

The treatments were painful. A needle was placed in my urethra (the pee hole) to shoot the medicine up into my bladder. I had to go through this treatment pain every week and often, in between, I had painful flares that made me go to the bathroom frequently.

Can you imagine sitting on the toilet for hours because you can't get up?

I.C. is a hundred times more painful than a urine infection (UTI). The lining of the bladder looks like a ball of fire from the inflammation. There is no cure for it. It causes depression because the pain can be unbearable, even with medications. This illness causes isolation and rocks relationships on all levels because of the intensity of pain and unfortunately, it also affects intimacy.

I was diagnosed in May 2008 and had enough of the illness by December 2008 (the pain started long before diagnosis).

I remember standing in my room and screaming out of pain to God to help me because I was done with this illness and needed an alternative. I was so fed up and angry that I threw away all the medications and everything that had to do with I.C.

My boyfriend at the time recommended fenugreek tea and oregano. I followed through. I also started to place my hands over my bladder and sent positive thoughts to her. I rocked her like a baby when she was in pain and spoke only kind words to her. Unlike before, when I'd get angry and wished for a new bladder.

My symptoms were relieved after only two weeks and took me about two years to be completely symptoms free. I also watched what I ate and focused on clean food. I reduced chemicals significantly from my life and drank herbal teas.

I say it took me about two years to recover or as the I.C. community calls it "to be in remission" because that's the last time I can recall a flare.

To further prove my recovery, I went back to the urologist in February of 2020 for an I.C. check and the doctor didn't find anything.

Another healing story:

When I was five years old, I had eye surgery for strabismus (crossed eyes). I hated myself for it and hated wearing glasses because I was bullied. After the surgery, I had to wear my glasses with brown tape covering my right lens. I looked like Jack Sparrow but worse. It felt awkward and I was embarrassed. The doctors told me I could stop wearing glasses by my teenage years, but then I would have to wear them again in my adult life.

I hated my glasses and had a strong desire to leave them behind forever.

As I was approaching my teenage years, I was able to stop wearing them by the age of fourteen. I had my eyes checked again at nineteen when I was told I don't need glasses, however, by the age of thirty, I should be prepared to start wearing them again!

At age thirty-five, I had my eyes checked once again and the doctor said my eyes are perfectly healthy there's no need for glasses! I believe it was my belief that I would not need them again that stopped me from needing them again.

The answer to the question whether or not we need healing modalities in order to heal is a yes and no.

The healing modalities are great to help you to create a connection with God/Source. It helps with developing trust. Trusting in God and in your body's ability to recover.

One healing modality I used while healing I.C was placing my hands over my bladder and sending love and positive thoughts to her. I didn't know back then it was a healing modality. Later on, I found out it was an ancient Hungarian healing method. In ancient Hungarian healing, we also bless one another the same way Christians do. Hungarian ancient healing believes that if a mother blesses a child, it provides great protection for the child. You place your hand over the head and from your heart, you say "God bless you"! You can do this with any pains as well and pray over it!

If you noticed most healing modalities come from ancient times like Reiki is from Asia and Aka Dua is from Atlantis.

In my years of experience facilitating healing for self and others, I discovered three components that are necessary for healing.

Making a decision

Creating the connection and trust in God
Follow through with divine guidance like clean food and herbs in my case of I.C.

1.   Making a Decision

You're the only one who can do this. I felt it in my heart and in my whole body that I was going to heal. This is something a facilitator can't do for you! Here we also get to calculate divine timing if God has a different plan for us, it must be honored.

2.   Creating connection and trust in God

This is where I truly believe the healing modalities are amazing tools. Your connection with God is everything. It was evident in my story of healing my eye as a child. I had trust in God, I was fearless and I knew anything was possible, so my doubts faded completely.

3.   following through with divine guidance.

In the case of the I.C., it was the herbs and food I ate that helped my healing. Later on, I did emotional processing to release emotions that were locked in my body because anger is a dark toxic energy. Also, food is medicine, so certain food recommendations can be divine guidance. I ate clean food, herbs and spices.

In summary, recovery is possible unless God wants something different. I wanted to heal and the most important thing was to make the decision to heal and align with Source, God, and the Universe. I started attracting people and situations that supported my healing. It's about trust and faith, to follow the steps for recovery!

Recovery is possible, freedom is in your hands!

Kinga Gecsey

Chapter 62

The Unknown in Healing

Some things are possible that we do not consider possible. I cannot say which helped me more, an openness within myself to what I previously thought was unlikely or impossible, or the use of healing modalities and substances like chiropractic, turmeric and ginger, or guided meditation and visualization techniques. But healing occurred beyond my expectations and beyond the viewpoint of highly respected medical professionals.

Three events in my life stand out when it comes to healing.

Healing 1. I had been working as a mason. One day I hurt my knee and was unable to walk without extreme pain. The doctor said I had torn a ligament or tendon and would need surgery, albeit arthroscopic surgery at first. I limped around with a cane for a while and then a few days before the surgery was scheduled a friend told me to see a chiropractor. I emphasized that I had hurt my knee so it did not make sense to go to a chiropractor who would adjust my spine.

But feminine wisdom can be very compelling so I followed her advice and went to a chiropractor who worked for the Boston Ballet Company. I asked if he could help my knee somehow. He said he did not think there was anything wrong with my knee, but I could try chiropractic for a few weeks and he expected that my knee would feel better. I figured I had nothing to lose so I tried it. I did not expect to get better and resigned myself to surgery, but found that I immediately felt better from the adjustments, and could walk easier. I postponed the surgery. Gradually my knee healed and never gave me a problem again.

Healing 2. I also suffered a work injury where I worked as a chef. I experienced extreme occasional pain in my right shoulder, which was revealed to be a SLAP (Superior/Lateral/Anterior/Posterior) tear on an MRI. This is when the ligament tears off the bone. The doctor said it was a partial tear. I said that sounds like good news because if it is only partial it can heal. They looked at me gravely with compassion as if saying, I do not think you are hearing us. The doctor affirmed that this was an injury that cannot heal without surgery, that it is not possible, as far as he understands. I said to him that it will heal by itself, and then I developed a healing regimen which included massage, chiropractic, turmeric and ginger in my diet, and supplementation with glucosamine, chondroitin and methylsulfonylmethane (MSM), as well as boswellia, omega-3 fish oil, evening primrose oil and borage oil, all reputed to be good for the joints. I also added olive oil, sunflower and safflower oil into my meals.

I did visualizations of healthy functioning in my shoulders, and guided meditations, while not overexerting or doing anything that would cause pain. This meant I predominantly used my left arm, leading to a SLAP tear in my left shoulder, from overuse.

The right shoulder had been getting better but now the left was out. Of course, I was disappointed and perplexed, but I was committed to healing and adjusted to the new injury with the same approach. I would even caress my shoulders at night and say I appreciate you and you are perfect and beautiful and resonating with your highest health and well-being and functioning. I spoke to myself and encouraged myself. And then I found a very fine holistic doctor, who agreed with the SLAP tear diagnosis, but did not recommend surgery and said it can heal over time if I do not re-injure it. This meant resting and no major, or even minor stress on the shoulders.

After several years of following my regime, both my shoulders healed completely. Now it is eight years later and I have not had any shoulder problems or pain. Although I am a bit careful, I work out, lift weights, dance and play and am active in ways that were not possible while I was injured, and rarely ever think about the injury.

Healing 3. At a certain time in my life, in my late twenties, I was very unhappy, and could not find a way out of what seemed like nearly constant inner pain. I was facing a great deal of personal sadness and confusion. I had gone to therapy for a few years and yet everything was still getting worse.

Finally, to heal extreme panic, anxiety, and an unreal amount of emotional pain I was prescribed medication. It relieved much of the anxiety, but my creativity, which has always felt like the most important thing in life to me, seemed to totally vanish. I also found that I put on weight, and though I am rather slim, my belly grew and I become rather heavy.

I kept feeling worse. I could not tolerate the feelings without the drugs, but I could not tolerate the drugs either. So, I decided to end it all. I had wanted to escape the immense pain for months and finally figured out how. I just had to go to the store and had it all planned out for a particular Saturday. However, when I arrived at the store it was closed, so I had to wait for Monday. I went to sleep, and then somehow got through Sunday, looking forward to the grace of Monday and the cessation of extreme suffering in which I felt there was no earthly way out.

On Monday I woke up and began to get ready to go to the store. Yet I noticed that I did not feel so bad. It was very strange and unusual, a complete surprise. As I went through the day, it amazed me that I did not feel the heavy deadening pain that had been a constant for many months. So, I figured that there was no particular rush, and postponed going to the store until the next day, when I expected the pain to return. Tuesday came, and again, no pain. After this went on for a few days, without any return of the intense pain I had been feeling all the time, I figured something had changed, and though I had no idea why, I was grateful, very grateful.

I became extremely grateful as the days went on, and the gratitude then shifted to joy, to immense joy and then states of bliss, unbelievable constant states of bliss where I felt as if I had just been born into paradise and everything was wonderful. My heart was full of love. However, this was interrupted by states where I felt dead, not intense pain, but it was heavy and uncomfortable. Yet, this would dissipate and I would feel relieved and better and then move into a state of joyful bliss again. The bliss deepened into what might be called transcendent ecstasy, and became more of a natural reality. It was quite remarkable. For a while, I kept going back and forth between these two states, until after about a month the dead feelings left, and the experience of high joyous ecstatic bliss became peaceful and constant.

People have speculated as to why this happened in such a way. They have said I am a walk-in, or that I let go inside so the pain left, or it was fate, or it was because of karma, or because I somehow invited God into my life, or that I believed so thoroughly that the pain would go away on a certain day, so it did. I have heard many ideas but as far as I can tell no one really knows, and that includes myself.

It seems that if we make way for mystery, for something to be possible which has seemed impossible, without reason, proof or logic, miraculous things can happen. And sometimes they happen anyway.

Somewhere along the way of surviving sadness and depression and realizing remarkably expanded beautiful states of being, I came to the spiritual insight that everything is joy. Everything in life is joy, ultimately, in its essence, including all experience. It subsequently became a great joy of mine to write poetry about these experiences and within these brilliant states of awareness.

William Michael Maisel

271

Chapter 63

From Allopathic Medicine to Essential Oils, Bringing My Boy Back from The Brink

There is something sobering about seeing your child hooked up to monitors, cannulated and lying naked and exposed in a hospital cot. When the expression of your love is not enough to take the temporal pain away, even if it is momentarily sufficient to keep him going.

When the medicine isn't working and he's not responding, what to do? When so-called 'professionals' do more harm than good and cause both physical and emotional trauma. When the prophylactic medications he's on to stop infections haven't worked. When he's not responding to the two sets of Intra Venous (IV) infusions he's on. When the three failed attempts to catheterise him have caused such internal damage to his urethra they CAN'T get the catheter in. When his temperature has hit 40.4 degrees centigrade and in addition to everything else, he is now having convulsions. When you are told that the emergency surgery he desperately needs to drain his kidneys is not possible and the risk of brain damage under general anaesthetic is too high...

What do you do?! What do you do when you have nothing left to lose other than your precious child? You do what any parent would do. You try ANYTHING - and you pray. This is when we shine our light, take matters into our own hands and where faith, belief and trust come into play. It would be easy to slip into darkness but then we remember that light casts no shadow, therefore we must emanate light and expel darkness.

You see my son, Arthur, has a super rare and chronic condition in his kidneys, found only the day before he was born and complicated by several 'kinks' in his ureter. If you'd have looked at his kidney scans from this time, they resembled far less kidneys and more so knuckle dusters. Just four huge, saggy VERY inefficient pockets.

His condition made him so poorly in the first ten months of his life. The longest stay we'd had out of the hospital and at home was six weeks as we were regularly transferred back to hospital with lights and sirens, on a weekly basis. It was always for a minimum of five days in hospital for a course of IV antibiotics. Six consecutive weeks at home only happened once in the first ten months and my goodness it felt incredible.

On top of this, my son had an operation every three months, to have a 'balloon' inserted into the base of his kidneys to try and stop them collapsing and then stents further down in an attempt to facilitate draining. They needed changing every three months to bigger ones as he grew. Imagine if you will, what a healthy kidney to bladder relationship looks like - a free-flowing stream of fairly clear water. Arthur's kidneys resembled more a stagnant pond of grot and grime, constantly filling and expanding his already weakened kidneys.

As a Reiki Master, Herbalist and Crystal Healer, I have always trusted and chosen natural medicine above all else. Arthur's High Dependency Unit incubator was always packed with crystals - much to the professional's bewilderment. Reiki was also regular, calling on my Medical Assistance Program as well as healer friends and colleagues too. I have absolutely no doubt that over the many times that he was on the precipice, these powerful healing modalities kept him earthside, however, he needed more and that's when I turned to essential oils.

The day described above was the day we were closest to losing him. He HAD to have his kidneys drained because they were going into failure. His temperature HAD to come down for that to happen. I set to work: peppermint oil on the soles of his feet - a cooling oil to help his temperature. Frankincense (the weaver of true magic) on my nipples before breastfeeding. Lemon oil in my drinking water and massaged across his kidneys for cleansing, clearing and detoxifying. On

Guard, a protective blend that is incredible for keeping infections, bacteria and viruses at bay sprinkled around his cot.

Within four hours of my beginning this regime, his temperature had dropped from 40.4c to 36.7c. He was taken off one set of IV's and the surgery postponed for observation after scans revealed his kidneys had 'miraculously' drained themselves. The medical professionals were stunned. We went home the next day. This was our shortest stay in Birmingham Children's Hospital, yet my son had been in the most critical condition. Both his surgeon and specialist urology team in shock.

He never did need that surgery. When we got home, I gathered all his allopathic medicine, including steroids and antibiotics and threw it in the bin. I was totally committed to keeping our home chemical and toxin-free, knowing that THIS would be the best support for my boy's kidneys. No vaccinations, nothing that was not natural in or on his body and probiotics and essential oils daily.

Arthur's mental and emotional scars took a bit longer, six months in fact:

Six months for him to grow in confidence enough to realise he didn't need to scream in angst every time a stranger approached him because they were no longer the nurses and doctors to who he was so accustomed to, doing uncomfortable and painful procedures.

Six months for him to get to know his big sister and Daddy really well after months of being apart.

Six months for him to let go of me and find simple joys in freedom away from the nurturing arms of Mumma and her boobies (thank GOODESS for boobies - the times they hung over a hospital bed comforting whilst needles were stuck in, bloods were taken and cannulas inserted. I salute you boobies and am eternally grateful!)

Essential oils changed our story and they have continued to work their magic and support him ever since. Even his scan pictures look different now. Don't get me wrong, medically he still has his condition but on a day-to-day basis it becomes easier and easier to trust the process of health, healing and wellbeing that his future will bring. I am proud of the courage, bravery and trust we displayed when we chose a more natural path for our son. A proactive one that cut chemicals and toxins out of our home to ensure we do all we can to support his kidneys, by means within our parameters to control.

In the four years since, I have supported hundreds of other people on their journey to wellbeing through the daily use of essential oils, either topically, aromatically and even internally. Reiki and essential oils create a symbiotic and powerful combination and I love to share them both with people to facilitate wholeness. If you would like to learn more, please don't hesitate to contact me.

Leah Napleton

Chapter 64

Healing My Sick Body with The Medical Medium's Protocols

My journey into becoming free of all my chronic symptoms and conditions started with the help of the Medical Medium books and divine knowledge. In just twenty-four weeks of following his protocols, some of my symptoms are almost a distant memory because of the huge improvements in my health.

My health problems started over thirty-five years ago. I was twenty-seven and pregnant with my last child. During the routine pregnancy check, the doctor noticed that I had cervical cancer. The doctor felt the best solution was to abort the baby and have a hysterectomy. I declined. I would carry the baby and suffer any consequences later as this baby basically saved my life by finding out I had cancer.

The treatment I underwent whilst pregnant was the freezing of the cancer cells, to prevent the spread during my pregnancy. After the birth of my son, I went in for testing and they could not control the cancer and sequentially, I had a hysterectomy. After that procedure, I was never the same. I started struggling with pain in my lower back and severe migraines. Over the next few years extreme fatigue, acne, bone loss, anxiety, swelling, eye floaters, guilt, memory issues, inflammation, spasms, neck and full chronic back pain, insomnia just to name a few things on top of the pain throughout my whole body.

I went from doctor to doctor with no relief. I was told that it was all in my head and became severely depressed, but I had to keep going as I had small children to care for. As the years passed, my conditions became worse. My life was difficult because the pain was so debilitating and intense. I was diagnosed with Ankylosing Spondylitis Arthritis (AS) and given steroids, which helped for a while.

After six months of treatment with steroids, the doctor decided I no longer had the AS and told me there was nothing wrong with me. I went to anyone I could find looking for any help; witch doctors, natural doctors, healers, Asian herbalist and had bizarre treatments. None of them helped and I still continued to decline. I would go days without sleep and the exhaustion would cause me to sleep for days, the pain was so intense I could barely handle it.

I was diagnosed with Epstein Barr Virus (EBV), Chronic Fatigue and Fibromyalgia. My loved ones did not believe I could feel that bad and that I was shirking my responsibilities. It would take every ounce of energy I could muster just to get through the day. I felt all alone and no one believed there was anything wrong. I was given prescriptions, one to wake up, three for pain, one for spasms, one for depression, one for sleep, weekly B12 shots, migraine medication and migraine shots. I became so depressed at one point I wanted to take my life. It's hell when no one believes you. I was barely existing. I would pray for strength to get through each day but the exhaustion was relentless. There were many, many days where I could not even get out of bed.

Fast forward another ten years; the daily migraines and migraine shots were brutal and made me violently sick. My pain grew more intense and I became so debilitated and bedridden. I could hardly move, let alone walk. Finally, I was seen by a pain management doctor who started a regime of medication. I started out with mild pain medications, spinal injections, injections in my head and quickly worked my way up to morphine. I was on strong opiates and steroids.

In all, five years of my life were spent being bedridden, on mattress island and not functioning. I begged for something to give me some relief as I knew I would die if nothing changed. I was dying, slowly, in my bed. As a consequence of being bedbound, I gained a lot of weight. I lost so much of my life to opioids and it is still too painful to talk about at the minute.

The doctor finally agreed and installed a pain pump with a mixture of medication to help me function with daily activities. I did get some of my life back but still suffered from chronic fatigue, insomnia, debilitating pain, migraines, cystic acne and bone loss.

Then I started having issues with my fingers turning purple in cold weather and the skin on my legs became very painful and purplish-black in colour. I went to numerous doctors, cardiologists and vascular doctors to no avail. Inflammation markers in my blood tests were off the charts and I was told to get it under control or it would kill me.

All the doctors and specialists I saw wanted to prescribed medication, but after suffering many nasty side effects of pharmaceutical medications, I declined and now wanted a holistic approach.

Doctors and dieticians made me sicker because of their lack of knowledge around nutrition and health. Disgusted with no help from any doctors, my daughter purchased the *Medical Medium's* (MM) books, *Secrets Behind Chronic and Mystery Illness and How to Finally Heal and Cleanse to Heal* by Anthony William. I was able to start working on MM protocols, started with celery juice. I drank twelve ounces daily and worked up to his thirty-two-ounce protocol.

Every other day, I had his Heavy Metal Detox Smoothie and the Liver Rescue Smoothie. I used his recommended supplements; B12, Zine, Lemon Balm, Nettle, Cat's Claw, Celery force, 5-MTHF, Barley Grass Juice, Micro C and did the morning cleanse. I cut out dairy, Starbucks, caffeine, meat and eggs and now only eat fresh fruit and vegetables.

I believe wholeheartedly that Anthony is an angel sent by God to answer all of our prayers. Anthony and the Spirit of Compassion have given us the tools to heal. Healing is possible. If you are serious about healing, please read his books, they have helped me enormously. I pray every night thanking God for Anthony and Spirit. I still have a long way to go, but I have come so far and I know that I WILL heal. I feel that for the first time in my life.

Major issues I dealt with every day, just to name a few:

- o   Cystic Acne
- o   Memory issues
- o   Cancer
- o   Anxiety
- o   Autoimmune
- o   Brain fog – severe
- o   Brittle nails
- o   Dark circles under eyes
- o   Eye Floaters

- Depression
- Swelling
- Extreme fatigue
- Guilt
- Hair thinning
- Migraines
- High blood pressure
- High Cholesterol
- Inflammation
- Joint pain
- Tinnitus
- Spasms
- Spider veins
- Reynard Disease
- Cysts

I think I have had almost every condition listed in the *Medical Medium* books. Yet, within twenty-four weeks of using his protocols, I can honestly say that the migraines, high blood pressure, anxiety, depression, memory issues and swelling are a distant memory. I have lost forty-five pounds and the other conditions I have are healing, slowly, so I'm still work in progress.

I know that Anthony William and Spirit of Compassion are the sources behind my glorious healing. I am very blessed and my gratitude will always be directed to them. They have given us the tools to heal. We just need to follow MM protocols, love ourselves again, start living life to its fullest and never look back. I am rising out of the ashes for the first time in thirty-five years and forever blessed and extremely grateful.

Ulla Escamilla

Chapter 65

"Manifest Who You Really Are!"

F irst, let me introduce myself. I am French-Canadian, born in Montreal, Quebec. Since I was very young, I felt that we had a lot of power inside of us. "All things are possible if you believe." I am telling you this because I know that to do our own healing there is a matter of faith, of absolute certitude in our capacity for healing. We don't heal at the level of doubt, only on the level of absolute certitude in ourselves. Also, the Universe seems to contribute when we really want something and when we do something about it for our highest good.

Myasthenia Gravis - Chronic autoimmune, neuromuscular rare disease: Muscles do not respond to the nerve command.

At fifty years old, I started to have a problem that manifested in my eyes. I started to see double which was very handicapping. It was like looking in a kaleidoscope all the time. The only time I could not see double was hiding one of my eyes with an eye patch. Doing this I lost the depth of my vision.

Besides the problem of double vision called diplopia, I had a nystagmus problem (involuntary eye movements), strabismus and ptosis (droopy eyelid). All this to say that I was not able to work for almost two years, of course, I was more dependant for some tasks. It took almost a year to get a diagnosis. During that time, I tried all kinds of things, including; acupuncture, visualisations, healing stones, etc.

I saw an optometrist, different ophthalmologists, surgeons and two neuro-ophthalmologists. I was finally sent to the Montreal Neurological Institute, where I had two tests, an electromyogram in my face and neck (about nine series of ten shocks) and another test introducing an electrode needle in my eyebrow. I accepted this torture because I wanted to have a diagnosis!

Finally, the neurologist told me "You have an incurable autoimmune disease, myasthenia gravis; if you are very lucky it will stay as it is but it should get worst. I had a young patient who died from this two weeks ago." Good news! I thought "I will heal, that's for sure!" At the time I did not know how but I knew for sure I will heal. Every day I was doing something in the direction of my healing, anything.

One day, I heard about a conference on "anti-gymnastic", I decided to go. It was very difficult for me to travel by bus and metro to downtown Montreal, in my condition. There I met a woman who saw that I had a problem and said to me "You know you can heal." I said "I know" … She replied "did you hear about "Décodage Biologique-Biologie Totale (Biological decoding - Total Biology)"? I said "no" and she gave me the name of a practitioner. I phoned him the next morning, started to work with him. I understood the root cause of my problem, took action and healed myself completely within few months, all this without any medication. I then took many courses and became a practitioner myself. This dis-ease has never returned, for the last eighteen years. The last time I saw the neurologist he told me "Yes, you are healed but it is not me who healed you...". I said, "I know, I did it with the tools of Recall Healing".

Breast cancer – cancer of the milk ducts or intraductal cancer:

Almost five years ago, after a mammogram test and an ultrasound, I was told that I had three nodules in my right breast. I then had a biopsy of the nodules and the doctors introduced three markers and I was told that I had "breast cancer".

I met the surgeon not long after who told me I had three choices, I thought I like the idea of having choices. He said: Aggressive chemotherapy / Surgery / Radiotherapy, in three different orders!!! I asked about the surgery and he wanted to take almost all my breast and suggested breast reconstruction. I said none of those choices, thank you. All I want is a follow-up. The doctors told me that if I did not accept the treatments I will probably die. I told them don't worry I am not a suicidal person and I know very well what I am doing. I had the chance to have the precious tools of Recall Healing.

Once again, I did the work I had to do to understand the roots causes of this. I was supported by some wonderful and generous colleagues. In the meantime, I did not stop my activities and on top of that, I renovated my house. Within about eighteen months, I was completely healed, without any medication. Of course, the doctors were completely stunned.

The precious tools:

I will try to give some clues here but you have to keep in mind that it is sometimes difficult to see our own conflicts because being blind about them is a subconscious way of protection, this is why we often need someone to help us to find information.

We are biological beings and the tools of Recall Healing are mainly based on biological laws. When there is too much stress the automatic brain will take over and send a program into our body. We can "deprogram" if we touch the right information. The right question(s) that caused a buried emotion has to come into awareness enough to be resolved.

Imagine an iceberg, the tip of the iceberg is your symptoms. The work I did, accompanied, was to find at the base of the iceberg the root causes, mainly with three ways: the events of the life (0 to now), what we call Project-Purpose (-9 months before conception / 9 months of pregnancy / +12 months), and the transgenerational conflicts (3 generations above). This work is about unlocking the secrets of illness.

There is too much to say here and I suggest you go and find some more information about Recall Healing. My friend and colleague Gilbert Renaud has also some videos in English to tell you more. Those two should help you to understand the basis of this approach, you can find some others on YouTube and also directly on the Internet site of Recall Healing.

https://www.youtube.com/watch?v=arHZHMmYgLk

https://www.youtube.com/watch?v=me09brGdDR8

If you need more information about my work and the tools I used, I will be happy to help you. In the year to come, I will have my own Internet site and will write a book. I practice in my home-office in Montreal and I am also on Skype.

As I say, those two dis-eases are part of the most beautiful experiences I had in my life because they contributed to help me be closer to Who I Am. I am happier since them and I realize how much it has helped me to understand the people I support and to be an example to let them know how powerful, how wonderful We Are and that Everything is Possible if we have faith, the absolute certitude and the right tools.

Hoping that my stories are inspiring you to keep going because what I did, you can do it. We are all made of the same essence, I am not the first one to be healed without any medication, there are so many others like Brandon Bays, Anita Moorjani, etc.

The greatest happiness is Being Who You Are!

Michèle Turcot

Recall Healing Practitioner

Chapter 66

My Healing Journey

My life-changing journey started nearly forty years ago (I am sixty-nine this year). I was exercising a horse for a friend. I did not know at the time that the horse had been shut in a stable for a while, resulting in me being thrown off.

That night my index finger was painful and swollen and I thought it might be broken from holding on to the reins. The next day the pain and swelling had travelled to another place and thinking this was odd, I went to the local doctor. She referred me to the Rheumatoid Arthritis (RA) clinic, whereupon I was diagnosed positive for RA and was consequently prescribed strong anti-inflammatory medications. I was later informed that as I was getting progressively worse, I would end up in a wheelchair!

Daily life became difficult and very painful, I carried on working and during the day the symptoms would get worse, so I would crawl up the stairs to bed as in a lot of pain. Suddenly, one day I could not talk and voices were getting more distant like I was not really there. My business partner immediately took me to hospital whereupon a young male Doctor declared that I was a neurotic female!

Fortunately, my partner had the foresight to take me to a private Doctor who, after extensive examinations informed me that I was suffering from side effects of the prescription drugs. I spent a very unpleasant three days at home, in a dark room detoxifying from the drugs and occasionally hallucinating.

The turning point came when a work colleague recommended a Radionics Practitioner that had successfully treated his wife for a chronic illness, so I contacted her. Radionics is a healing modality that measures and analyses vibrations, through a client's hair or blood. A programme of different frequencies then targets infected areas and brings the body back into equilibrium. Body parts have their own rhythm and balance and when dis-ease sets in, this rhythm and balance become distorted which is detected by the machine. Skilled practitioners are then able to analyse, measure any distortions and identify the cause of the problem, i.e chemicals, bacteria and parasites.

The human body responds in a similar way to a radio/tv and becomes a receiver of the prescribed frequencies and starts the healing process to rebalance the body function.

We are all connected through the electromagnetic energy field of the earth, so clients don't need to be present as their hair or blood is sufficient. I continued with this treatment, having daily contact by telephone with the practitioner, keeping her informed of any symptoms I was experiencing and she would make adjustments to my radio frequencies. This continued for a period of three months until I reached the stage that all the symptoms were gone. I could even straighten my hand which was becoming quite deformed.

The local doctor had not heard from me in a while, so summoned me to her office to discuss operating on my hand. When she saw that I had healed it and after I explained what had happened, she struck me off because I had refused to follow her advice!

This experience changed my way of thinking. The drugs I had been prescribed were later withdrawn from the market due to adverse side effects. I started doing my own research and joined the "What Doctors Don't Tell You" group. I started studying homeopathy, herbalism, nutrition, naturopathy, holistic medicine, pH balancing, healing mind and body therapies and bio-pulsed magnetic therapy.

I occasionally experienced repeat swellings in my fingers, so I went along to a well-known Naturopathic Clinic in London and was advised to go on an elimination diet for one month at a time, starting with dairy products and then wheat, but to no avail.

I thought the swellings could be from eating and drinking oranges as I was consuming quite a lot. After eliminating them completely for one month, the swellings stopped completely. Just to test my theory, I drank a glass of orange juice and the symptoms returned. My gut feeling was correct.

I became interested in the acid/alkaline balance of the body and I used the PH testing sticks (dipped in my urine) to measure acidity levels in order to avoid arthritic symptoms. My reading was six (a reading of between 7 to 7.45 is a good balance). I made adjustments to my diet avoiding acidic forming foods. In some people, orange juice has an acidic effect on the body.

My interest in bio pulsed magnetic therapy came through fate. My horse became spasmodically lame and I found a therapist who lent me her battery-operated bio pulsed magnetic machine. After treating him for three months, my horse was healed. Bio pulsed magnetic therapy applies pulsed frequencies to induce small electric charges in the target tissue, aiding the body to heal and regain normal functioning. The applicator pad is applied to the injury, two or three times a day and the pulse rate is altered accordingly till the healing is complete. I was so impressed by the machine that I purchased my own and used it to heal my fractured ankle and my husband's ruptured Achilles' tendon.

After my horse died, aged thirty-two, I started S.E.A.R.C.H, the Spanish Equine Association for Rescue Care and Homing / *Associacion Española para rescate y adopcion de Equinos*. I rescued a five-year pony with a badly broken shoulder. Dr David Somerville the inventor of the bio pulsed machine kindly sent me the latest model, adapted for horse use, as a gift for the Charity. After a course of treatments, the pony is still with us ten years on, loving life.

I became very sick at the end of my second summer in Spain and could not eat, barely move and had a high fever. In desperation, my husband called a local Radionics practitioner who came to the house and hooked me up to what is commonly known as a 'zapper' machine. It sends out mild electric waves that 'zap' parasites and bacteria in the body. The radionics practitioner continued to work on me from home using a sample of my hair as a medium and daily telephone calls to monitor my progress until I was fully recovered.

Following this illness, it left me with a predisposition to pneumonia/bronchitis and lung problems. I use a breathing device called an AIR PHYSIO, similar to an asthma device but chemical-free and designed to exercise and expand lungs to expel mucus, a saltwater and aloe vera nasal spray and drink homemade, herbal teas, to manage my own health and wellbeing.

I went on to develop and make my own healing cream initially for the animals to treat sores, bites, irritations that can quickly otherwise become infected in the summer heat and also to keep vet bills down. It proved so effective that my family now use it and I give it to other charities and people in return for a donation for my own Charity and is known as the 'miracle cream' by users.

I believe that my destiny was triggered by that fateful day I fell off the horse and that everything happens for a reason even if it seems bad at the time. After it, my life went in a different direction. I now teach students to work with horses, using body language and energy with the ultimate aim of achieving a telepathic connection. This has resulted in life-changing experiences for many students.

To be healthy, we need to concentrate on our lifestyle, exercise, nutrition and thoughts, turning negative ones into positive ones. Your life is in your hands. As Captain Sir Tom says, 'tomorrow will be a good day'.

Susan Barns

Chapter 67

TEN Tips for Self-Healing from Toxins and Heavy Metals

I have been on a long journey of healing from leaky gut, heavy metals and candida. My usual symptoms are a sick tummy and a feeling as if all my energy is draining through a hole in my body.

Diet is always the first place to look. I use a restricted Paleo with no grains, legumes, or nightshades which has really helped and eliminated all processed sugar and packaged products. I use herbs; comfrey or lemongrass for tea and eat fruit in small amounts. The fats I use are olive or coconut oil and butter. The Gut and Psychology Syndrome Diet (GAPs) is also a good diet to start supporting the body.

One of the issues with molds and heavy metal like mercury, is the inability of the body to get these toxins out of the body. When I'm having a 'flare', I spend a lot of time in bed sleeping and/or meditating. My brain doesn't function well, and my body has only the energy for essential things. If I'm too ill to get dressed, I'm not able to drive to a store.

When I'm looking for solutions, they need to be easy and readily available. These are my solutions.

1. **Rest and Breathe**: To assist the healing process.

When I'm unable to sleep I use meditation to focus on any pain in the body and bring light to this area.

I give myself permission to rest when I need to, I read a book or play a game without guilt.

2. **Meditate:** Meditation can change the body, bring peace and wholeness.

I use a Yoga Nidra (Rest meditation), to relax. Sometimes just music, sometimes guided.

There are apps available to use, or make your own meditation guide.

3. **Soak in a Bath:** This moves the lymph to get toxins and metals out of the body.

Ionic Foot Baths have copper cores and use salt water to create a field to pull the lymph out the feet. One session elevated my mood and energy.

Epsom Salt soak in a warm tub, I don't have a soaking tub, so I just soak my feet in a tub of Epsom Salt water, after doing a Bentonite Clay Foot Detox (see recipe below).

4. **Sauna:** I have an Infrared sauna but if my body is too weak for this and I can't get my body to sweat, I'm only bringing up more toxins that I cannot release.

Dry Brushing before a sauna helps me to produce more sweat.

5. **Clay as a binder, to carry the toxin out of the body:**

Bentonite Clay - (food grade) used externally or taken internally

Neolite Clay - used internally; a very fine soluble clay that assists detoxification.

Chlorella and Spirulina also help bind and remove heavy metals; however, I react to both of these with a rash, possibly due to iodine.

6. **Marijuana** - assists with nausea and relaxes the body and mind. Smoking tends to make me very tired so I limit the THC amount and the usage.
7. **Energy Work**

Tibetan Tonglen Energy Healing purifies the energy in the sick body. I did this for two cats and my horse and noticed an increase in their wellbeing, so I have written a Self Tonglen Meditation (below) that I use, with good effect.

Reiki healing sessions clear and cleanse my energy. I either do it myself or with a trusted practitioner.

Sound - Tones from voice or bowls can break up and release illness. However, I find that tones can be too much if the pain or illness I have is acute.

8. **Stones** – Ask permission of a stone or crystal to absorb pain or sickness. They are eager to assist and enjoy the experience.

I sit with the stone on my body or cupped in my hands, keeping my awareness on the sensation in my body, and let that energy flow to the stone. Be sure to thank the stone afterwards!

9. **Essential Oils** - Only use pure oils

I use a diffuser to get the oils into the air for improved air quality and to help the body.

Lavender is a good all-round oil to have on hand. Healing for burns, anti-fungal, anti-viral, anti-bacterial, and is safe for cats. There are many oils to choose from.

Raindrop: This is like a massage in the application by a trained practitioner;

I have done a 'mini-raindrop' for myself which helps relaxation, and purifies the body's cells. Like other detox modalities, you have to be able to pass the toxins out with water. So, this isn't recommended for heavy metals.

10. **Water** - Water water water

Purified, or filtered from the tap, I drink half of my body weight in ounces for maintenance. When ill or detoxing, I double or triple it!

Shungite is a carbon-based stone that helps with EMF blocking. I put it in my water for beneficial results, along with clear quartz crystal.

First thing in the morning, I add one tablespoon of freshly squeezed lemon juice or apple cider vinegar to my water.

Bentonite Clay Foot Detox

Half a cup Epsom Salt
2 Tbsp. Bentonite Clay
1 Tbsp. Apple Cider Vinegar (ACV)
6 Quarts Very Hot Water

In foot basin; combine hot water and salt, set aside

In a glass bowl mix clay and ACV together. Coat the bottoms and tops of the feet with clay mix. Let sit for ten minutes to dry.

Soak feet in the foot bath for fifteen minutes, the clay will dissolve and fall away.

Rinse feet and dry off

Self Tonglen Meditation

This is an Energy Meditation that will take you through releasing energy and purifying it before returning the purified energy to the body.

Ground and center your energy; above, below and North, South, East and West

Imagine a "bag of holding" resting before you that you will place energy into.

Start at the base of the torso, place your attention at the base of your spine. Breathe slowly and rhythmically and be aware of the body and any sensations.

Intention - I allow any past or present patterns to flow easily and comfortable out of this area and into my bag of holding in gratitude, acceptance and love

Move to each area of the sacral, solar, heart, neck, back of the head, third eye (pineal gland), and crown of the head, resting in each position for at least three breaths setting your attention and stating the intention at each area to easily move energy to the bag.

Place your attention on the 'bag of holding'.

Intention - I call on my Higher Self, guardians and guides to receive with thanks this energy and ask that this energy be purified in love.

See a white light from above pour into the bag, shining and overflowing with radiant angelic love. Observe any colors or sensations quietly.

Intention - I welcome this purified energy with gratitude and love easily and comfortably into my Self.

See the bag of shining energy returning into your body and welcome the spreading of this love energy throughout your body. Then rest and breathe, your attention is on love, peace, wholeness, perfection of this light within and without all the cells of your body.

Pamela Means

Stone Dragon Energy
Spiritual Technical Guide
Certified Aromatherapist, Raindrop AND REIKI Practitioner
Young Living Essential Oils & LifeWave Distributor

Pain

"The strongest people are not those who show strength in front of us but those who win battles we know nothing about"

Unknown

Chapter 68

I am Healing, Inside and Out

In Summer 2018, I was diagnosed with Post-Traumatic Stress Disorder (PTSD) following a traumatic incident. Between extreme noise sensitivity, depressive thoughts, insomnia and night terrors, life had become a struggle at home and at work. A few months later I badly hurt my ankle, severely injuring the nerves, leading to the development of Complex Regional Pain Syndrome (CRPS). This was on top of anxiety, Irritable Bowel Syndrome (IBS) and a history of depression. CRPS is a chronic pain and nerve disorder that is higher on the McGill pain index than amputation or childbirth. The onset of CRPS was thought to be connected to the PTSD, for after all, the body keeps the score.

At first, CRPS confined me to a wheelchair and/or crutches. On a cocktail of pain-relief drugs, I completely lost my mobility and was in pain twenty-four hours a day, seven days a week, unable to even wear socks or shoes. Almost all the strategies to manage PTSD, through undergoing trauma focused Cognitive Behaviour Therapy (CBT), went out the window with most of them being physical.

Wanting to get better

The first step in my healing journey was a desire to get better. Despite what the doctors told me, and the fact that I may never recover, part of me wanted to improve (even if a full recovery wasn't possible). Following the initial diagnosis, I was referred to another specialist. I even invested in a private appointment with an orthopaedic surgeon as I didn't feel like I could wait another six weeks to have the diagnosis confirmed. An MRI scan was done confirming the diagnosis. After my own research online, I learnt that experts say that the chances of CRPS healing are higher early on, so I knew I needed to advocate for myself and put pressure on my doctor and the medical staff. I started having physiotherapy, and then argued massively for hydrotherapy as it had helped me immensely with a previous ankle injury in 2014 and many sources online stated it as important for CRPS treatment. I then started connecting with others with CRPS on online forums and found out about a specialist centre for CRPS in Bath. I knew I had to go there, liaised with my doctor, and saw specialists there who gave me more recommendations to heal. These included desensitization therapy, psychotherapy - specifically Eye Movement Desensitization and Reprocessing, (EMDR) for trauma, reducing stress levels, and strength building through physio and hydrotherapy. I felt seen there for the first time and was told I was doing everything right...but I continued to be mentally and physically unwell.

Investing in myself

The second step, early in 2020, was investing in myself, putting my healing and wellbeing first. Not only did I really put into practice recommendations from the CRPS service, but I read online medical articles, educated myself, and the big one...prioritised my health, in a holistic way, above all else. I finally stopped trying to balance a full-time job with all my medical appointments, exhausting myself in the process and despite my fears, changed to part-time hours, three days a week, as my organisation agreed on medical grounds and the medical professionals were concerned with the hours I was working.

I continued psychotherapy and fully devoted myself to it, reading self-help books, developing a regular self-care practice as well as learning and setting boundaries. I learnt how to say no, and tackled embedded perfectionism. I committed to meditating, even when calming the mind felt like the hardest thing in the world, developing a daily practice over months of striving. I got myself back to yoga, even before I couldn't walk, seeing it as an opportunity to both de-stress and to strengthen muscles.

I started seeing the osteopath regularly to look after my full body. I self-massaged my ankle every day (sometimes three times a day) using a Chinese trauma balm. I used a heated foot spa every day. I took supplements; vitamin C and magnesium. I continued physiotherapy both at the hospital and also at home. I continued my hydrotherapy exercises both at the hospital and on my own at the local pool. I then began swimming once I was able to, even if it was a length or two. I paced myself, increasing my steps on nearly a weekly basis, working my way up from the post-box at the end of the street to walking into town about a mile away. I invested in a personal trainer to strengthen my muscles and lose all the weight I had gained for being immobile for many months. I started eating better.

I began healing the trauma symptoms, by going to EMDR therapy, which was one of the hardest things I've done, uncovering a whole series of events prior to the trauma episode, that had made me feel unsafe. I connected with the "spoonie" community on Instagram. I advocated for accessibility rights. I grieved the loss of my mobility. I continued the pharmaceutical medications and then worked up the courage to reduce them little by little, over a period of time, working with my doctor. Gradually I went from two to one crutch and onto a cane. For a while, I was sure that was the extent of my recovery, as progress became so slow, it was almost difficult to see.

Believing I could heal

In August 2020, I came across Sarah Harvey's free twenty-one-day healing programme with the Self-Healers Society; meditations, journaling prompts and resources. It is through this program that I finally came to the revelation that "I get to heal". The crazy thing is that I did not even realise that on some level I was unconsciously blocking my own healing. Somewhere deep inside me, I did not believe that I could heal. Maybe it was because the doctors told me that my diagnoses were chronic, maybe it was because I didn't believe I was worthy of healing or maybe in some way being sick served me. Maybe it was all of the above. Through this programme, the membership, and one-to-one coaching, I was able to recognise all this, then choose not to believe any of that anymore. Instead, I choose to believe that our bodies have an innate ability to heal ourselves. I learnt also how words matter and stopped identified so much with "my pain" or "my CRPS", rather referring to "the pain" or "the symptoms". I also learnt the importance of self-compassion.

Since summer 2020, I have continued to heal, my symptoms are slowly but surely lessening. I no longer walk with a cane. I can now lift certain things. Since early 2021, I have been able to come off all forms of meditation, taking only now CBD oil for pain once a day. I can shower standing up without aid. I am more physically able, and I am in a better space mentally. I am shifting my mindset, letting go of what no longer serves me and creating a life more in alignment with what does.

For me, this means, amongst other things, training to be a yoga teacher to support others in their healing and recovery, guiding meditations and sharing my story.

I am doing the inner work, challenging my thought patterns, actively choosing to soothe my nervous system and healing inner child wounds.

What does life look like now? I meditate daily. I practice yoga. I see a physiotherapist regularly. I work with a personal trainer. I eat well. I listen to my body and my mind. I swim regularly. I have a nourishing morning routine that serves me. I journal. I express gratitude. I trust the universe.

I am healing, inside and out.

Abbie Huff-Camara

Self-healer, yoga teacher and meditation guide.

Chapter 69

Chronic Pain Healed with A Positive Mental Attitude and CBD

Many moons ago, in 1998, to be exact, I had a normal job and a passion for dogs that is still with me today. Back then I had four and one of them, Woody, was a very longhaired shaggy boy who needed a groom regularly and in summer loved nothing better than to be shaved. One Sunday afternoon I settled in for the task with my grooming kit and clippers. Three hours later and the task was complete. By the following morning, my hell had begun!

I awoke in the morning to walk the dogs and head off to work only to discover my right arm was swollen and I could hardly move it. It was agony. In those days I used the national health, as did anyone, and ventured off to the doctors. I was diagnosed with repetitive strain injury and possible carpal-tunnel syndrome for which I would need a hospital appointment; go home Miss Wood, two weeks off work, and don't use it! Pain killers, anti-inflammatories. A bit of a shock and actually not possible with four dogs, but of course did my best and awaited the appointment.

During my time off I noticed that the other hand was also hurting but put that down to grooming my Woody. I also had neck and upper back pain, again, down to the grooming.

A few weeks later I had the appointment and after tests, X-rays etc I was diagnosed with carpal-tunnel syndrome and then the big one, Ankylosing Spondylitis. The pain by now had become unbearable and so was given far stronger pain killers and sat back to watch it slowly progress to a point I could hardly move. The hospital informed me that the only option was morphine and amitriptyline for the pain, then I was prescribed more drugs to stop the sickness that went with the concoctions of drugs. I knew I had Hypothyroidism (an underactive thyroid), so had the drugs for that, but slowly everything was becoming too much.

I degenerated pretty quickly and began to lose feeling in my hands and could not bear any changes in temperature. I could hardly move my hands. The next and only option I was told would be surgery on the carpel tunnel, they also decide that the nerves were in a bad way and would operate on the elbows as well, allowing more mobility after the operation recovery time.

The decision was made to do each arm at a time which would mean no mobility of the arm for a long time afterwards as it would be in a plaster cast and then once removed, physiotherapy. By now I am basically zonked out and in a different world, one I certainly did not want to be in. I was signed off as disabled as nothing functioned and my work entailed lots of computer work.

The first arm they did was the left and it was bloody awful! I had to let it recover enough that the cast was off and the arm was usable before they commenced with the other. A few months later, they did the right and it only confirmed that the left was much easier. I had to learn to write all over again, the pain was incredible and of course, to alleviate this there were so many drugs it was ridiculous.

I was now at the point of sitting most of the day, I could do nothing through the pain and not having a clue where I was with the drugs. So many days I no longer wanted to be here.

All this was over a period of four years, my employers after negotiations and doctors' reports that all confirmed that I would no longer be able to work, certainly not for a period of less than five years, gave me early retirement, which saved my sanity and the stress, but now what?

My last appointment at the hospital was to discuss the spine and they said my only option was an operation, they could not guarantee it would help, or that it would even allow me to walk properly and there was a slim chance it could go wrong. Aaarrgh! No chance, they were not touching my spine, never! So, what now? I was told go to somewhere warm and enjoy what I could as I would be in a chair within two years.

That day, and after discussions with my then partner and friends the house went on the market, once sold, the decision was made to come to Spain.

Sold my home, came to Spain a whole new life beckoned and yet the drugs continued. I registered with the Spanish system and went regularly for check-ups and was always sent home with a huge back of drugs, all pain killers in some form. Nothing was improving and my relationship crumpled, so now I was alone and no idea what to do.

It became slowly worse until I was on so much morphine for the pain it affected the rest of my body and my mind; I had no choice but to return to the UK.

I returned with my brood and rented a lovely railway carriage on the Solent, Isle of Wight, continued my treatment with the hospital but now the damage had been done, my bowel had failed due to the stress and my liver and kidneys were in bad condition; I had a Hiatus Hernia and the drugs and stomach acid had destroyed my stomach. Again, I was offered a plastic reconstruction, more surgery and I refused. I was panicking and no idea what to do, but through another relationship, amazingly I returned to Spain, this time in the campo, where the weather can be very hot and dry during the summer months. So definitely warm then!

I was still taking the drugs, which now include statins for high cholesterol, God knows how, apparently hereditary. What a mess!

Now comes the part where suddenly life is put into perspective and you realise that if you don't do something, no one else is going to and my whole life, thought structure and self-care began.

I somehow followed my dream of saving dogs and other animals, opened a rescue and sanctuary, called Barkinside, absolutely wonderful. My heart and soul were filled with joy and passion. Somehow, I stopped thinking or feeling the way I had, I also knew, there was no way I could continue the work in the condition I was in and with all these drugs in me. You have to be quick, strong and on the ball, there had to be another way.

I had heard, through the internet and friends talking about CBD oil, so researched what turned out to be my truth. I found and made a dear friend who guided me through everything and started very slowly, introducing it to my body over a period of time. I began meditation, reading, being calm, being grateful and full of joy, leaving negativity and anyone who brought that into my life. Rescue is incredibly stressful so these rules had to apply. I still use the CBD creams and lotions and use it on the dogs as well. It has changed many of their lives.

Every month my health improved and I slowly reduced my tablets, a massive step. You need to be as fit as you can be, mentally and physically to do this job and now after five years, this has changed my life. I only take an antihistamine, yes I am allergic to dogs! The levothyroxine for my thyroid, which I cannot stop and omeprazole for the heartburn, which to be honest I get if I overindulge and we are all allowed to do that from time to time. I still feel the cold and my hands hurt, so I wear finger cut off gloves.

I do not take one pain killer and I absolutely refuse to. I have not seen a doctor in the eleven years I have lived here on my return and I have been running the rescue for six years.

Your life can change, take that step, take hold, be all you can be, never give up.

Jacqueline Roberts

"Barkinside Dog Rescue"

Chapter 70

Healing Complex Regional Pain Syndrome

t's quite fascinating, the mind-body connection. Since March 2019, I suffered from various health problems. I had debilitating leg and foot pain and ended up in a wheelchair on two occasions because I couldn't walk. I was put on multiple medications, none of which helped and in fact my health declined further. Doctors believed all my problems were all caused by a herniated disc.

By the middle of September 2019, I had received two separate nerve injections and had undergone two surgeries on my back. After the second back surgery, I had to use crutches for almost two months. My mental health suffered due to the constant pain I was left in and the feeling of being abandoned by the medical system after my neurosurgeon said: "it's just pain". I believed it was part of their job, to help relieve pain.

I was basically left with a diagnosis of Complex Regional Pain Syndrome, CRPS, for which the Doctors say there is no cure. I was also told that it is an autoimmune disease and "it will spread, possibly to your organs and attack them".

I had to learn how to heal myself as the Doctors didn't think it was possible. However, I proved them wrong because I have healed about ninety-eight percent now (from the last wheelchair hospital incident October 25, 2020, when I couldn't walk again and I was sent home with pharmaceutical medications).

I found out how to heal by addressing the trauma stuck in my body. I was able to learn through various reading, podcasts, research and techniques that I found regarding the mind-body connection.

The techniques I focused on were; self-hypnosis at bedtime and repeating mantras with breathwork through the pain flares. I also did do some Emotional Freedom Technique (EFT) tapping.

I continued to push through the pain with exercise originally to slow the dystrophy (wasting) and spread of the disease. I started with small knowingly achievable goals and kept pushing past them over time. My five thousand steps turned into ten thousand. I also had to slow myself down at times and give myself a day of rest because occasionally, I was over motivated. The "why" in healing needs to be stronger than the "why not."

My diet changed and I removed gluten, dairy and meat but kept eating fish because Omega 3 fatty acids are an anti-inflammatory. I also started taking supplements and herbs to support the gut-brain connection.

I'm a very outdoorsy person so I refused to accept I would not be able to go into nature because I know being outdoors in green spaces really helps improve mental health. I went out for walks on my crutches, not an easy undertaking. Persistence is key to remind the brain and body what normal sensations feel like.

I did things to laugh and play with my inner child through creative outlets. I worked on my emotional pain and trauma, which is a big issue in chronic pain or illness sufferers.

I had to raise my spirituality and vibration with inspiring stories of hope and recovery in people who had extreme diseases like stage four cancer, to reaffirm the placebo effect. The heal documentary is a great resource of inspiration.

The medications I was given for chronic pain caused me side effects that I didn't like. I had an allergic reaction to Gabapentin so it was changed to Cymbalta, which sent me into a deep depression with anxiety. I weaned myself off the medication and then through withdrawal. That was when I reached out, looking for non-pharmaceutical alternatives. Self-hypnosis helped me overcome the numbness from the medications. I had to learn to interrupt the fight or flight response and used breathwork and mantras. I underwent a complete lifestyle change.

After being abandoned by my Doctors, I contemplated suicide a few times because of the helplessness I felt and the pain I was in. I tried talk therapy but it didn't work for me or for the trauma I had gone through. I understood that I needed to be focused on the emotions I felt, to be able to release the pain I was constantly in.

I used a punching bag to release my anger and negative emotions. I soon found that my positive emotions returned, especially with my repeated mantras of self-worth and self-love and self-compassion, to shut down my inner critic. I had to remove the inconsistent programming of unworthiness.

Recovery isn't a straight line, so I expected relapses of pain. In understanding this, I found it made them easier and faster to overcome.

Neural reprogramming was one of the big factors in my healing. It is basically extinguishing the old pain pathways that had been developed and reinforced over years, and replacing them with newly created ones, of healing and not of fear around pain. Pain is our internal alarm system to pay attention to our emotions. It's truly a gift. People also need to understand the pain is real but the origin is from our unconscious mind. It's amazing and difficult all at the same time. It is literally a system reboot and is truly one of the miracles of mankind!

People have been believing in a magic cure through medication and invasive procedures because they have been told so by medical Doctors, but there is no magic cure. We have to take responsibility for our own recovery and when we do, miraculous things begin to happen over time. We don't know how long it may take because our illness didn't just happen overnight.

My mind healed and I had new ideas; I am energetic and healthy. I feel like I had to reboot my mind and body, as you would do to your computer. It's a gift you can give to yourself.

Sacheen Collecutt

Poisoning

*"The wound is the place
where the light enters you"*

Rumi

Chapter 71

Healing Botulinum Toxin Poisoning

My name is Maria Bajo and I am a survivor of the cosmetic product, Vistabel (Botox) made by Allergan, administered during my treatment from 11 March 2008 to 02 October 2009.

Over the last ten years, I have had many telephone conversations and reports done, regarding my case. The only advice Allergen gave me was to go to the emergency room. I was left alone to figure out how to heal, suffering from the severe side effects of Botox. During this period, I felt like I was dying and visited doctors many times.

The side effects of Botox include at least fifty different types of symptoms including heart problems, difficulty breathing, vertigo, brain fog, acid-burn feeling in the brain and all over the body, losses of consciousness, anxiety, sleep attacks, memory loss, loss of speech, extreme fatigue, loss of bladder control, depression, extreme fear, jerking and shaking, panic attacks, paralyzed feeling, numbness, sensitivity to flash lights and noise, dizziness, teeth decay, depersonalization, fainting feeling, hallucinations and joint pains.

The doctors in the UK informed me that there was no cure at this horrific advanced stage of poisoning and time would heal. My recovery gradually started about five years after the injections were administered.

Six years after the original treatment, I began to see the light at the end of the tunnel. It's now been ten years and I have not recovered fully. To my dismay, I have subsequently developed new symptoms which worry me, as the majority of people poisoned by Botox develop autoimmune diseases, like multiple sclerosis and cancer. This has had a devastating and damaging impact on my life and career.

CAREER: I have begun to make progress in my career again. I finally finalised my dream project, a fitness DVD last year.

CHILDREN: I remain childless at forty-seven years old because I suffered from Botox poisoning during the time I was planning to have children with my partner at that time. Instead, he became my caregiver because I was so ill and as I started to recover, he left me.

FINANCIAL LOSS and HARDSHIP: My recovery took all my savings.

During my first five years of recovery, I contacted many professionals and patients who appear to have a connection with Botox use: doctors, scientists, Botox victims, survivors, Allergan, Hungarian National Institute of Pharmacy and Nutrition (OGYEI), Hungarian and UK media.

I visited many doctors to seek their knowledge and opinion about my situation. The pain, brain fog and acid feeling all over my body and brain, heart and breathing problems have been intense, every minute of every day, for years. At times I was on the verge of going to Switzerland to a euthanasia clinic.

Dr Anna Hristova examined and diagnosed me with iatrogenic (relating to a medical treatment) botulism. I am one of the case studies in her paper about Botox: Impaired Neuronal Communication Syndrome as Novel Neurological Side Effect to Botulinum Toxin Type A Therapy with 16 Case Reports.

Dr Sandor Rideg, a well-known Hungarian neurologist, detected the parts of my brain where the poison had settled and where it attached to the nerve endings, using a German method. He recommended a natural healing route, over pharmaceutical medications.

Dr Sarah Hart is a spinal specialist and her thermographic scan showed the blockage of the central nervous systems which prevented the free flow. She scanned me three times and I was treated by her for four years. The scans clearly show the effect of Botox poisoning. Many of the victims had the same scan and we all had the same results.

Dr Oliver Cockerell has many clients who suffer from iatrogenic botulism and told me that there was no cure, only time would heal it. Some recover but some never do.

Dr Matteo Caleo wanted to see the stage and how the poison affects the myelin sheath. He confirmed that at the time I saw him that Botox was undetectable in the body.

Dr Ella Kukier has already detected the Botox poison in a few victims' blood in the past two years and she said that within two to three years from the injection time the poison is usually detectable with her method. She agreed to test my blood even though it had been six years. The results shocked everybody.

Dr Cockerell's theory is that the poison will eventually be covered by cell tissue, which can be activated any time by any action, so the poison itself isn't present in the blood anymore. However, Dr Kukier detected forty types of ingredients and proteins which are used only for Botox cosmetics.

Six years after my original injections, my blood and body are still full of foreign bodies which can cause serious autoimmune reactions and cancer in the future, confirmed by Dr Sharla Helton and other doctors. This is evidence that the injection does not stay in one place and the reason that I still have relapses and light symptoms. My body and immune system are still fighting to clear the foreign cells, proteins and spores. Dr Sharla Helton will provide many studies in her research, proving that those foreign ingredients cause more damage.

I can work part-time now, but my life is still challenging. I do my best to stay away from any medication and drugs as I don't want to poison my body further. Since 2008, I have not had any medication, not even a painkiller. Medications should be used only for saving lives in emergencies.

My recovery journey has involved only using natural remedies, raw food, oils, herbs and some vitamins. I found which foods negatively impact the immune system and stopped eating them.

As soon as I was told that I suffering from Iatrogenic Botulism, I started researching and contacting people who had anything to do with Botox. After I learned that the poison goes into the brain and affects the nervous system, I did much research and focused on how to heal my brain.

I highly recommend living a life without any medication unless is very much needed. Thank you for the opportunity to able to tell my story and to help and encourage others to live a life without medication.

Maria Bajo

KANGEN WATER DISTRIBUTOR

FITNESS, LIFE-STYLE AND HEALTHY LIVING ADVISER, PT,

REFLEXOLOGIST, REIKI HEALER

GROUP EXERCISE INSTRUCTOR

Co-Founder/Producer of Fitness to BoneyM Tunes 60 min exercise program. Watch our 60 second Promo to our new fitness DVD on YouTube

Chapter 72

Healing from Family Poison

I come from a predominantly toxic family which has the constant of three generations with neglected "inner children" that live inside "adult bodies".

In the year 2017, I was living at my aunt's house: someone who had both lupus and fibromyalgia. At this point, I was preparing to embrace my path more truthfully and she became the perfect exploration field of the "emotional cause" of illness, despite the ongoing emotional triggering that came with her guilt-tripping and constant manipulation for everyone to bend their will towards her, I was able to see first-hand the conflict within that was causing her to "cast upon herself" two chronic autoimmune disorders.

Living with my aunt, I noticed a chain of behaviors and events that led to her conditions becoming chronic. From my observer point of view: my aunt was filled with resentment, her eating habits were filled with self-punishment, she hated to cook but when others cooked for her it was never good enough and she always had a negative remark to conclude a positive one and so on.

After almost four years of living with my aunt, her negativity finally took a toll on me, a toll that would manifest in 2018, right after leaving her house and moving back to my mother's house.

I had a natural distrust for doctors and people with "white robes" as early as my younger years and my fascination for medieval times was already paving the path for the untapped potential of Gaia's cabinet (nature's pharmacy). My inclination towards holistic medicine started at the same time as my spiritual awakening, ten years ago. At first, it was a curiosity: I would google the benefits of fruits and vegetables I was eating.

Jumping back and forth through the years and depending on my situation, I went from vegetarianism to "eat whatever people offer me" and started harnessing an internal GPS when it came to foods that weren't bringing me wellness.

It all started with a meal that left a bad after-taste. On this occasion, my mom had cooked one of her overly seasoned meals that I immediately rejected. I ended up eating it because there came the shame, the guilt-tripping and the nagging. My body, however, wasn't very happy about it. It was starting to pile up resentment both from my previous housing experience as well as the revival of much childhood trauma regarding control at my mom's house. A few hours into ingesting the meal, I started to feel a bloat, a bloat that turned into a fever and leading to "I think I may not make it out of this one".

I felt my liver swell after a few hours, then the fever started, the shivers followed, I started vomiting and couldn't hold onto any food or liquid. My mother amplified the condition by fueling me with her "pharma" fear, dosing me unwillingly with Tylenol (Paracetamol) and Pedialyte (electrolytes). I felt worse and worse each day.

Fevers are a way in which our body uses "raising our temperature to kill any potential pathogens" by the way. My mother, being a firm believer in "people with white robes" and google medical symptoms 1 to 100 and therefore started her fear campaign on me shortly after the second day. I still had a fever. This is when the shivers began, I had intense shivers and she kept freaking out, which as an empath only put me in a more depleted state of mind. She would sit on the edge of my bed in an exacerbated state of mind reading all symptoms to me as I was ready to check out: "Laura, you could have hepatitis right now, look at this and that, oh my god, oh my god, oh my god."

On the fourth day of what felt like me going in and out of my deathbed hours, I gathered some strength to make my voice heard: "leave me alone, I will do what I need to do for myself, I know what my body needs".

The night before I had started going over my knowledge from the book of herbal facts, in my mind and intuitively felt resonant with CBD oil and Milk Thistle. Milk Thistle detoxifies the liver and CBD oil has anti-anxiety, anti-inflammatory and calming properties.

I was working up an intense "food poisoning" scenario but it was more than that, it was also a resistance to my environment, to being controlled, to feeling oppressed, to resenting the beliefs I had been brought up with which contradicted my holistic ways, just because "they are family". What was family anymore, if the moment you disagree with them you are cast out? All of these questions were important self-talking points as I battled the rage of the fever that expressed itself through my liver and onto my whole body.

Looking like a corpse, I went to the local shop and bought myself CBD oil and Milk Thistle. I also found an Indian recipe to clear the liver. It contained; aloe vera, ginger, lemon, black salt and was to be consumed every few hours. That same day, after starting my natural regime, my fever died down, I was able to go to the bathroom not to puke and I could breathe again.

In the days that followed, I added lots of fresh greens, cilantro, fresh fish and light salads to my diet and I drank lots of hibiscus tea. It was a rebirth like no other and one of my greatest proofs of my naturally inclined convictions and the potential our bodies have to fire the codes of self-alignment.

I also have to admit that my confrontation with my mom, was also a pivotal part of my healing as it was the moment I got my power back about my own choices, no longer conditioned by her fear as I had lived most of my life. Healing is ultimately a third-dimensional process of deep integration and your body is just waiting for your command to restore itself.

My aunt, on the other hand, had taught me the greatest lesson of all, with her resistance to healing herself by not wanting to even acknowledge all her pain and the pain she was inflicting in others for not validating herself ever. This solidified my posture when it came to illness, knowing what I knew then, I could ALWAYS heal myself. Had I not believed this from my research years before, I would have never had the will to pursue it.

Laura Piquero

Chapter 73

Healing A Severe Adverse Reaction to Vaccines and Dengue Fever with Plant Leaf Infusions

---

I honestly don't know how to start my story but first of all, I am very happy to be part of this book and honoured to share my story with the world. I am Oni Abayon Estillana, but please call me Jodie as this is my nickname. I am thirty-six and a Filipino.

Four years ago, I was studying a caregiver course and to complete our course we had to undergo on the job training. We were not allowed to proceed to the on-the-job training in a hospital until we had the Hepatitis B vaccine.

Our clinical instructor said that everybody must have two shots of the Hepatitis B vaccine, to protect us from the viruses in the hospital and to boost our immune system.

From being a child, I always remember my father had told all my family that we should never receive any vaccines. This is because he believes we can all heal ourselves in natural ways, so I was very scared. However, I didn't have a choice. I had to take two shots of the Hepatitis B vaccine to enable me to finish my course. So, despite my worries, I had the shots and had to pay for them too, 1,500 pesos in our money.

Just a week after my month's training in the hospital, I was very sick. I was so ill that I couldn't move my body. I had a high fever, pain and a rash all over my body, but particularly bad on my chest and legs and I did not know why. I knew it wasn't anything I had eaten as I can eat everything, except pork, which is not allowed because of our religion. My family are Seventh Day Adventists.

I was really worried at this time and started questioning myself about why I had suffered when I had the vaccines. I was told they would boost my immune system so why did I get sick?

I didn't go to the hospital at this time because I didn't want to be sick in a hospital. I stayed home and took care of myself. My friend was concerned about my health but I told them I could recover at home by taking natural remedies to lower my fever and staying hydrated, drinking lots of water.

After being sick and virtually bedbound for two weeks, I was able to stand again and walk on my own, so I believed that my life would be normal again. However, I now had searing pain and felt like I was going to die because it was so bad. I got myself through this period with a lot of self-will and determination.

After I had recovered, I started researching vaccines. I had no idea what was happening in the world of vaccines. I realised that I had suffered from a severe adverse effect of vaccines. I was so shocked when I realised that they contain so many toxic ingredients and they had poisoned my immune system. After more research, I found out how to detoxify myself and started by drinking herbal infusions made from medicinal plants and leaves, mixed with hot water.

I used the leaves of lagundi (Chinese chaste tree/five-leaved chaste tree/horseshoe vitex), guava, Guaynabo, mango, sambong, pandan (screwpine) and apatot (cheese fruit/Indian mulberry/wild pine), as well as ginger and drank them daily.

These leaves were used fresh, after being rinsed thoroughly and cut up into small pieces and sun-dried then boiled. But please note; sambong, pandan and apatot are not good for pregnant women because they can cause miscarriage.

I drank these infusions every day. I also drank coconut juice with raw egg. This is not only delicious, but it is good for cleansing inside.

As I am religious, I prayed every day that God will return my strength and heal me fully.

Vitamin Sea is also a great healer of pain, wherever that pain is in the body. I swam in the ocean every day because we live near to the beach. Swimming in the ocean and walking on the beach helped heal the pain in my body. I also laid on the sandy beach, which helped heal my pain too.

Any time I have pain, I go to the beach with my sister and the pain disappears. It's like magic.

Dengue Fever

Recently I suffered from Dengue Fever. During this time, I only drank water and infusions made from tawa-tawa (snakeweed) leaves as well as the extract of papaya leaves. It's very bitter but really effective for dengue fever.

Bed rest is a must and I ate a lot of quail eggs. Drinking at least two raw eggs in a day is really helpful to normalize the platelets.

When I tested positive for dengue fever, I was really worried because I hate to be in the hospital or have any vaccination like Dengvaxia. There has been a big scandal here in the Philippines and many children have died because of the Dengvaxia vaccine.

I'm so thankful to the Lord that he created those natural medicines in nature for everyone and for every sickness we have. The only thing we must do is to research and ask anyone who might know the answers to our questions. Never hesitate to ask anyone you think could help you especially the older people who know mostly everything regarding natural herbs. And of course, as a Christian believer, always trust the Lord that nothing is impossible, so please ask him to help.

I am still doing my research on vaccines and talking to many people to learn more. I share this knowledge with others who don't know. Some believe me and others are sceptical. I know a time will come everyone will enlighten their minds, especially when the dengvaxia scandal that happened to our country is known.

Drink herbal leaf infusions for healing. If you have an instinct about something, never ignore it.

I hope this can helps others too.

Oni Abayon Estillana

Chapter 74

From Living with a Medical Blindfold to Light and Knowledge: Saving My Vaccine Injured Brother with Natural Remedies

Over the years I slowly leaned more toward natural remedies versus pharmaceutical because it's partially in my blood and a big part of a huge learning process. You see I have a vaccine-injured disabled brother. He is two years younger than me. He was born in 1980 in soviet Armenia and because of the time and the regime we lived in, he was damaged by vaccines and medical malpractice yet no one was held accountable!

Fast forward to 1998 when we moved from Armenia to the USA. My brother was evaluated re-diagnosed and put on multiple psychiatric medications and he started attending a few different programs designed for people with similar disabilities.

Fast forward another ten years or so: due to his injury and the combination of the medications he was on, he developed ulcers that almost killed him. He was hospitalised for a while where he contracted scabies. For those who don't know what that is, scabies are colonies of microscopic bugs under your skin that cause unimaginable itching hives and discomfort.

This was a huge ordeal for myself and my family, from start to end. We had to learn how to heal from the toxic medications we had to use to get rid of the scabies themselves.

Long story short, I had to go back to basics and relearn what I know about healing both skin and internal organs naturally.

I turned to oils and that's where I discovered the amazing healing powers of oils, essential oils, simple carrier oils like coconut oil and even CBD and cannabis oil. I learned about natural remedies for pain and inflammation and how to heal the gut after being on medications for a long time.

This helped my brother a lot, as a matter of fact, it was the key to his healing. I used to have to mix many oils to put on his tortured skin after finally getting rid of scabies. It was the best thing for him, helping him heal and recover. I used CBD and cannabis oil to heal his mind and psyche.

My brother went through a huge trauma of severe autism and brain damage as a result of vaccine injury. At one point in his illness, he was close to death.

We used many detox baths to help him push the toxins out. We also helped him to heal his gut with diet and probiotics. With the help of natural remedies and diet and lots of love and help from God, he made a full recovery!

That's my story and I hope it inspires someone to give natural remedies a try.

Araksia Enezliyan

Part Three

"Nothing is impossible. The word itself says I'm possible"

Audrey Hepburn

Afterword

Following my healing journey and the collating of other's healing journeys for this book, I truly understand that for us to heal, we need to address not just our physical needs, but also our mental, emotional and spiritual needs too.

Mental

This is our thoughts, attitudes, beliefs, desires, values, and goals. These can be crucial in determining what we experience as symptoms. We can improve our mental health through meditation, mindfulness, education and goal setting.

Emotional

This is about connections with ourselves and others. As we reconnect with our emotions through mindfulness without judgement, we can bond with our lost inner child. Practising self-reflection, gratitude and forgiveness strengthens our emotional needs.

Spiritual

This is about our connection to energy, our true essence, our oneness and understanding that we are all connected. Often it is us, ourselves, that are out of alignment with our spirituality. Being conscious and present in the moment, practising mindfulness and prayer all support our spiritual needs.

Physical

A healthy physical body is gained through:

Nourishment – eating nutritious foods and drinking natural beverages

Gentle exercise – walking is great and very undervalued, outside in green space is the best

Sleep – around seven to eight hours of uninterrupted sleep

Breathing – a daily practice of deep and slow breathing

PLUS – all the other needs being met and in harmony, as our physical body is a reflection of our mental, emotional and spiritual bodies and needs.

Sadly, modern western medicine doesn't appear to take a holistic approach to health and seems to focus only on the symptoms rather than the root cause of dis-ease. This book highlights that often, the root cause is a mental, emotional or spiritual issue, manifesting real physical symptoms in the body. Therefore, as we heal our mental, emotional and spiritual bodies, our physical body heals.

Much dis-ease today appears to emanate from unresolved traumas, often from when we were small children. For us to heal ourselves, we need to undertake some inner work, to resolve this trauma. As we forgive ourselves and others, for not having the skills needed to deal with the situations which occurred, we start to let go of the hurt we have held onto, often unconsciously. In forgiving and letting go, we are not forgetting, rather we stop holding on to it and carrying it around with us and we start to heal our physical symptoms.

Our body is healing, every day. It's what it does but often, we just do not see what is going on.

The Mind-Body Link

The mind-body link has been proven by many, with the placebo effect highlighting how our mind can create healing; so, if it can create healing, why could it not create dis-ease? Can we accept that it is plausible then for our body to be manifesting what our subconscious mind believes, therefore we are co-creators of our suffering?

So, if we have co-created it, surely, we must be able to heal it, right? Absolutely, if we can just believe we CAN heal and believe that we are WORTHY of healing. It is about our belief in our belief.

The healers in this book are testament to the fact that natural self-healing IS possible.

May you be blessed with the belief in your belief of healing.

Much love

Sarah

List of Contributors

Below is the list of all the wonderful self-healers who have contributed to this book, organised alphabetically by their second name, along with their contact information where given. Please note that where someone has preferred not to give contact information, I have noted this. Please respect each individual choice.

I cannot thank each and every one of these wonderful people enough for being a part of my journey to bring this book to you.

Oni Abayon Estillana
No contact information

Maria Bajo
Email   maria.bajo@btinternet.com
Facebook   MSfitnessLondon

Rebecca Barker
No contact information

Susan Barns
Website   www.serch.es

Christine Barrett
Website   www.healjoyfully.com
Instagram   @healjoyfully

Susie Berns
Website   www.simplebalancetoday.com
Email   Susie@simplebalancetoday.com

Joana Bonança
Website   www.fromhivtohealth.com
Facebook   fromhivtohealth

Kim Boutelle

Website	www.holisticwellnessbalancedlife.com
Email	kimboutelle@ymail.com
Facebook	Holistic Wellness Balanced Life

Mila and Steven Bromley

Website	www.HondonValleyHomes.com

David Brown

Facebook	davidmatthewbrown3
Instagram	@unabashedyogi

Patrick Cave

Website	www.patrickcave.com

Kim and Kay Cherry

Website	www.alswinners.com

Sacheen Collecutt

Email	elephant.training@outlook.com

Patricia Dickert-Nieves

Website	www.TheMultipleSclerosisCoach.com

Paul Dumper

Website	www.arcwellbeing.com
Facebook	arcwellbeing

Petra "EatJuicy"

Websites	EatJuicy.com
	GreenSmoothieGangster.com
You Tube	petraeatjuicy
Instagram	@petraeatjuicy
Facebook	petraeatjuicy

Araksia Enezliyan

Email	araksia_e@yahoo.com
Facebook	roxyartsy818

Ulla Escamilla
No contact information

Carolyn Evans
Website   modere.com.au/?referralCode=144484
Email   rpcievans90@gmail.com

Heidi Foster
No contact information

Kinga Gecsey
Email   gecseykinga@gmail.com
Instagram   @kinga_holistic
Facebook   KingaGecsey

Laurie Graham
Moringa web link   healthy-mind-healthy-life-with-
laurie.isagenix.com/
Email   Simply.scentered@hotmail.com
Personal Facebook   laurie.mitchell.9216
Instagram   @LAURIE_GRAHAM75

Tina Hakala
Website   www.sacredrootsholistic.com

Teresa Harris
Facebook group   The Transitioning Vegan

Sarah Harvey
Website   theselfhealerssociety.com/membership
Instagram   @iamsarahharvey
Podcast   Not So Chronic

Kaylene Hay
Website   www.kaylenehay.com.au
Facebook   Kaylene Hay – For the Love of Self

Smitha Hemadri
Web	www.smithahemadri.com
Instagram	@smithahemadri

Jane Hogan
Website	www.janehoganhealth.com
Email	jane@janehoganhealth.com
Facebook	janehoganhealth
Instagram	@janehoganhealth
YouTube	janehoganhealth
Pinterest	janehoganhealth
Linked In	jane-hogan-5609b83a

Bonnie Hoo
Website	www.bonniehoo.com
Email	daringtoconnect@gmail.com

Sigrun Hornberger
Website	www.RavenWolfMetaphysics.com

Susan Horwell
Website	www.susanhorwell.com
Email	susanjhorwell@gmail.com
Instagram and Facebook	@thehealingtableuk

Linda Hoyland
Website	www.lindahoyland.com

Abbie Huff-Camara
Instagram	@abbies.healing.corner

Grace Hughes
Website	https://linktr.ee/EarthboundSerafine

Stephanie JoyousMind
Website	joyousmindhealing.support
Email	stephanie@joyousmindhealing.support

Donna Kilgallon

Email	donnahomoeopath@gmail.com
Facebook	DonnaKilgallon
Twitter	@DonnaKilgallon

Angie Kim

Website	www.angieguidesyou.com
Instagram	@angie.guidesyou
Facebook	Angela Kim

Fania Koh

Website	www.missionfeelgood.com

Alex Korosec

Facebook	Alex Korosec

Yvette Laboy

Website	www.yvettelaboy.com
Email	coachyvettelaboy@gmail.com
	inspiredwellness@yahoo.com
Instagram	@coachyvettelaboy and @fromlupustoliving
Facebook	CoachYvetteLaboy
YouTube	Yvette Laboy Lupus Wellness Coach

Jill Law

Email	jlaw1951@hotmail.co.uk

Jenny Levine Finke

Website	www.goodforyouglutenfree.com
Instagram	@goodforyouglutenfree

Vanessa Lewis

Website	www.vanessamariaaromaterapia.com
Email	vanessamaria2012aromaterapia@gmail.com
Facebook	vanessamariaaromaterapia
Facebook	OilsforlifeSpain
Email	oilsforlifespain@yahoo.com

Bonnie Madrigal
No contact information

William Michael Maisel
No contact information

Melissa Marson
Web   www.Melissamarson.com
Email   support@melissamarson.com

Diana Martin-Gocher
Website   www.Thrive-DianaPhD.com

Dawn McCrea
Website   energyhealingstrategies.com
Facebook   EnergyHealingStrategies

Pamela Means
Email   meansp@mtaonline.net

Karina Melissa
YouTube   youtube.com/karinamelissa
Instagram   @karinaxmelissa
Twitter   @karinaxmelissa
Email   karinamelissa13@gmail.com

Jojo Mohr
Website   www.homewithjojo.com
Email   mohryogawellness@gmail.com
Instagram   @homewithjomohr
Twitter   @JojoMohr

Gaylyn Morgan and Thomas Runte
Website   www.gaylynmorgan.com
Email   Gaylyn@etnur.net and Thomas@etnur.net

Marcia Murphy
Email   marciainasheville@gmail.com

Leah Napleton
Email   info.essentoillyu@gmail.com

Kathy Newman
Websites	www.amazinglifebalance.com
	www.fyihappy.com
Facebook	AmazingLifeBalance
Instagram	@amazing.life.balance
Twitter	@KathyNewmanALB

Samantha Nicole
Website	www.leveluphwh.com
Email	leveluphwhcoaching@gmail.com

Raymond Patrick
No contact information

Ashley Pharazyn
Website	www.myquainttraditions.com
Facebook	ashleypharazynhealthcoach
Instagram	@my.quaint.traditions

Laura Piquero
Website	https://lpmylott.wixsite.com/lauraswritingstore

Tripat Riyait
Instagram	@inspire.calm

Jacqueline Roberts
Website	www.barkinside-dogs.com
Email	barkinside69@aol.co.uk
Facebook	Barkinside

Consuelo Robles
Website	www.casalabodega.com
Email	concienciarte@gmail.com
Facebook	consuelorobles

Julie Rose

Website   www.dorsetholistichealth.co.uk/

Website   JulieRose449289595.arbonne.com/

Website   credenceonline.co.uk/shop/

Danielle Sims

Instagram   @daniellesimswellness

Kevin Smith

Facebook   Abslike300

Instagram   @ib3kevin

Domenic Stanghini

Website   www.dstanghini.com

Kristina Stephenson

Website   www.mygeneticsonline.com

Stephanie Stewart

Website   stephstewarthealing.com

Hazel Stinson

Instagram   @hazel_stinson.wildly_healing

Lucia Stone

Email   mexicolucia@gmail.com

Facebook   Lucia Stone Canales

Alice Taylor

Email   alicetaylor3@hotmail.co.uk

Alexander Thermos

Website   www.LifeSourceWellnessCare.com

Email   sandra@lifesourcewellnesscare.com

Michèle Turcot

Websites   www.recallhealing.com (English)

                  www.icbt.ca (French)

Email   turcotmichele@gmail.com

Skype	Healingbyrecall

Rachel Turner

Website	www.rachelturnerwellness.co.uk
Email	contact@rachelturnerwellness.co.uk
Instagram	@rachelturnerwellness
Facebook	rachelturnerwellness

Index of Health Issues

A

B

C

D

E

J

K

L

M

N

O

P

R

S

T

U

V

Glossary of Terms

Acne – a pimple that develops deep in the skin, causing a red, swollen, and painful bump, can be hormone related

Acupressure – is acupuncture without the needles, instead using manual pressure from the fingers

Acupuncture – a Traditional Chinese Medicine (TCM) technique of stimulating specific points on the body by inserting fine needles through the skin

Acupuncturist – the person doing the acupuncture

Adaptogens – a select group of herbs that support the body's natural ability to deal with stress

Addison's Disease – a condition in which the adrenal glands do not make enough of certain hormones

Adhesions – bands of scar tissue that binds two tissues together

Adrenal glands – small organs located above the kidney which produce and release several hormones in the body. During chronic stress, the adrenal glands produce less of the hormones needed to feel healthy

Akathisia – a movement disorder, inner restlessness, unable to sit or stand still

Alternative medicine – the practice of medicine without the use of pharmaceutical drugs

Anaphylactic shock – a life threatening medical emergency from a sudden and severe allergic reaction involving more than one body system

Anemic/Anaemic – the lack of enough healthy red blood cells to carry adequate oxygen to the tissues of the body

Ankylosing Spondylitis Arthritis (AS) – a form of arthritis that primarily affects the spine

Antacids – medication used to treat excess stomach acid

Antibiotics – medication used to kill bacteria

Antibodies – proteins produced by the immune system in response to an infection

Antihistamines – medication used to treat allergic reactions

Anti-inflammatories – medication used to relieve pain by reducing inflammation

Anxiety – an emotion characterized by an unpleasant state of inner turmoil and nervous behaviour

Aromatherapist – a person who provides holistic medicinal treatments through the topical application or inhalation of natural oils

Asthma – an inflammatory condition of the lungs in which the airways narrow and may produce extra mucus. Symptoms include wheezing, breathlessness, chest tightness and coughing at night and/or early morning

Atherosclerosis – a disease caused by the build-up of fats, cholesterol and other substances on the walls of the arteries, which can restrict blood flow

Aura – a field of energy

AuraChakra healing – healing the chakras and auras and improve life

Auricular therapy – a technique of stimulating points on the skin of the outer ear

Autism/Autistic Spectrum – a disorder of development characterized by difficulties with social interaction and communication

Auto-immune – an abnormal immune response to a functioning body part

Autonomic Nervous System (ANS) – a control system that mostly acts unconsciously and regulates bodily functions

Ayurveda – a form of holistic medicine that focuses on promoting balance between the body and mind

Bach flower remedies – flower essences derived from wild flowers, plants and trees that correspond to specific emotions

Bee venom therapy – the therapeutic application of honeybee venom, through live bee stings, to bring relief and healing for various conditions

Beta blockers – pharmaceutical medications that are used to manage abnormal heart rhythms and reduce blood pressure

Bile – a liquid that helps break down fat from food

Bioenergetics – a way of understanding personality in terms of the body and its energetic processes

Biological decoding – finding the conflicts associated with behaviours and diseases as well as the relation to each organ and system of the body

Biological laws – diseases are age-old biological special programs of nature, created for our survival

Biopsy – a sample of tissue taken from the body in order to examine it more closely

Black box warning – an alert for serious side effects, such as injury or death

Boil – a pus filled, infected hair follicle

Botanical – of or relating to plants or plant life

Botox – an injected neurotoxin, used for medical and cosmetic purposes

Brain fog – diminished mental capacity marked by inability to concentrate or to think or reason clearly

Brain-Derived Neurotrophic Factor (BDNF) **peptides** - a protein produced inside nerve cells to help brain health

Breathwork – any type of conscious breathing exercises or techniques

Brucellosis – a bacterial infection that spreads from animals to people

Buhner protocol – a holistic treatment protocol developed by herbalist Stephen Harrod Buhner, using three herbs and five points of philosophy

Bulimia Nervosa – an eating disorder characterized by binge eating followed by self-induced vomiting

Caesarean section – surgical procedure used to deliver a baby by cutting open the abdomen

Cancer – the uncontrolled growth of abnormal cells anywhere in the body

Candida – a fungal infection within the mouth, gut, vagina or penis, caused by yeast

Cannulated – having a hollow tube into a vein, for the administration of liquid medicinal products

Carpal Tunnel – a condition that causes pain, numbness, tingling, and weakness in the hand and wrist from the compression of a nerve

Cataplexy – sudden and transient muscle weakness that occurs while a person is awake and triggered by strong emotions

Catheter – a thin, flexible tube that can put fluids into, or take them out of, the body

CBD Oil – a naturally occurring compound found in the flower of a cannabis plant

Celiac Disease – an autoimmune condition causing severe damage to the lining of the small intestine, triggered by gluten

Cervical (spine) – neck

Cervical cancer – a type of cancer that occurs in the cells of the cervix, within the vagina

Chemotherapy – an aggressive form of chemical drug therapy meant to destroy rapidly growing cells in the body that can have severe adverse effects both during the therapy and for some time after

Chikungunya virus – an infection that causes fever and severe joint pain

Chiropractor – trained doctors who specialize in detecting and reducing misalignments of the spine

Chronic Fatigue Syndrome (CFS) – a debilitating, chronic disease that affects the nervous system, the immune system, and the body's production of energy

Complex Regional Pain Syndrome (CRPS) – excessive and prolonged pain and inflammation following an injury

Cold laser trans-cranial therapy – low-intensity laser therapy that stimulates healing, using low levels of light

Colitis – inflammation of the inner lining of the colon

Colonic – involves flushing the colon with fluids to remove waste

Colonoscopy – a procedure to look at the inside of the colon, using a flexible tube with a camera

Constipation – bowel movements that are infrequent or hard to pass

Convulsions – an episode of rigidity and uncontrolled muscle spasms with altered consciousness

Corpse – a dead human body

Costochondritis – inflammation of the cartilage in the rib cage

Counselling – giving guidance or therapy

Cranial Sacral Therapy – a system of very light touching to balance the craniosacral system

Cyst – noncancerous, closed pocket of tissue that can be filled with fluid, pus, or other material

Dandruff – a condition that causes the skin on the scalp to flake off

Dengue Fever – a mosquito-borne infection that can lead to a severe flu-like illness

Depression – a mood disorder that negatively affects feelings, thoughts and actions

Dermatologist – a doctor who manages diseases related to skin, hair and nails

Detox/Detoxification – the removal of toxic substances from the body

Diabetes – insulin production is inadequate or the body has become resistant to insulin

Diarrhoea/loose stools – loose, watery and bowel movements/stools

Disk – shock absorbing structures between the bones in the spine that allow movement

Distant-healing – energy-based healing sent to others not in close proximity to the healer

Diverticulitis – a condition of inflamed pouches/pockets in the lining of the intestine

Double vision – the seeing of two images of a single object

Dry brushing – the process of brushing dry skin with a long-bristled brush

Dystonic reactions – repetitive or twisting movements caused by muscles contract involuntarily

Ear infection – infection caused by virus or bacteria in any part of the ear

Eczema – a condition that causes the skin to become itchy, dry and cracked

Ehlers-Danlos Syndrome (EDS) – a group of genetic connective tissue disorders. Symptoms may include loose joints, stretchy skin, and abnormal scar formation

Electroencephalogram (EEG) – a test to evaluate the electrical activity in the brain

Emollient creams – creams, lotions, or ointments that contain ingredients that soothe and soften the skin

Emotional Freedom Technique (EFT) – a form of acupuncture that uses the fingertips to stimulate energy points on the body, also called tapping

Empath – someone who picks up on the feelings and emotions of others

Encephalitis – inflammation of the brain

Endocrinologist – doctors who specialize in hormone related diseases of the endocrine system, a system of glands and the hormones they make

Endometriosis – tissue similar to the lining of the uterus grows outside of the uterus

Energetic body scan – a machine to measure the energy wavelengths of the body

Energy work – used to help balance the systems of energy throughout the body to alleviate stress, ailments, and disease

Epigenetics – the study of how the environment and other factors can change the way that genes are expressed

Epstein Barr Virus (EBV) – a common virus that causes mononucleosis/glandular fever

Essential oils – compounds extracted from plants that capture the plant's aroma or essence

Eye floaters – small spots that drift through the field of vision

Eye Movement Desensitization and Reprocessing (EMDR) – a trauma focused psychotherapy

Fasting – relating to the abstaining from food but can also include fluids

Fatigue – a feeling of tiredness or lack of energy

Feldenkrais – a type of exercise therapy to reorganize connections between the brain and body to improve body movement and psychological state

Fibromyalgia (FM) – a debilitating, chronic condition that affects the nervous system, the immune system, and the body's production of energy

Fissurectomy – a surgery used for curing anal fissures

Fissures – cuts or tears in the tissue inside the anus

Folate – the natural form of vitamin B9 in food

Folic acid – a synthetic form of vitamin B9

Follicle Stimulating Hormone (FSH) – a hormone that stimulates the ovaries in women and the testes in men

Gall stones – pieces of solid material that form in the gallbladder

Gallbladder – an organ that stores bile

Gastro-intestinal/GI/ Digestive tract – the tract from the mouth to the anus which includes all the organs of the digestive system

Glandular fever/Mono – a viral infection caused by the Epstein-Barr virus. Symptoms of fever, sore throat, fatigue, and swollen lymph nodes

Glutathione pushes – Intravenous therapy of glutathione (antioxidant), given over fifteen minutes

Gluten – a family of proteins found in grains, including wheat, rye, spelt, and barley

Glycaemic Index (GI) – the ranking of carbohydrate in foods according to how they affect blood glucose levels

Gratitude – the expression of appreciation

Graves' Disease – an autoimmune disorder that causes the thyroid gland to create too much thyroid hormone in the body

Gynaecologist – a doctor who specializes in the health of the female organs

Haematologist – a doctor who specialises in the diagnosis, treatment and prevention of diseases of the blood

Hallucinating – having sensations that appear to be real but are created within the mind

Hashimoto's Thyroiditis/Disease – an autoimmune disorder that can cause an underactive thyroid

Hay fever – Inflammation in the nose as a reaction to allergens in the air. Symptoms include a runny or stuffy nose, sneezing, red, itchy, and watery eyes, and swelling around the eyes

Headache – pain in any region of the head

Heart attack – insufficient blood supply to the heart causing damage or death of the heart muscle

Heart coherence – using the power of the heart to balance thoughts and emotions to achieve energy, mental clarity and feel better

Hepatitis B – a liver infection caused by the hepatitis B virus

Herbalist – a person specialising in the therapeutic use of plants to prevent and treat illnesses, promoting health

Hiatus hernia – a condition where the upper part of the stomach pushes up through the diaphragm into the chest

High blood pressure (Hypertension) – the pressure of blood in the arteries is persistently elevated

Histamine – a chemical released by the immune system in response to potential allergens

Hives – a form of skin rash with red, raised, itchy bumps

Hoist – equipment to lift and transfer a person with limited ability from one place to another

Holistic – dealing with or treating the whole of something or someone and not just a part

Homeopathy – the practice of natural medicine that embraces a holistic approach to the treatments

Hormone Replacement Therapy (HRT) – a treatment for women with low hormone levels

Hormones – substances produced by the endocrine glands that effect bodily processes

Hot flashes/flushes – a feeling of intense warmth and/or sweating, lasting a short duration and related to hormone disturbances

Hyperbaric Oxygen Chamber – a pressurized tube that provides pure oxygen at greater than normal atmospheric pressures

Hyperemesis Gravidarum – an extreme form of morning sickness that causes severe nausea and vomiting during pregnancy

Hypermobility – the ability to move joints beyond the normal range of movement

Hypersensitivity – a state of altered reactivity in which the body reacts with an exaggerated immune response to a foreign agent

Hypnosis – a mental state of highly focused concentration, diminished peripheral awareness with heightened suggestibility

Hypnotherapist – a person who induces a hypnotic state in clients, to alter behaviour patterns

Hypochondriac – a condition in which a person is excessively and unduly worried about having a serious illness

Hypothyroid – a condition in which the thyroid gland is not able to produce enough thyroid hormone

Hysterectomy – an operation to remove a female's uterus

Iatrogenic – harm to health caused by a healthcare provider or medical treatment or diagnostic procedures

Immune system – a system of cells, organs, proteins, and tissues that work together to protect the body from infections

Immunoglobulins – an antibody used by the immune system to identify and neutralize bacteria and viruses

Inflammation – a response triggered by damage to living tissues and a normal part of the body's defence to injury or infection

Inhaler – small, portable, hand-held devices that deliver medication to the lungs

Insomnia – a sleep disorder that causes difficulty in falling asleep, staying asleep, or both

Intention – a mental state that represents a commitment to carrying out an action in the future

Intermittent fasting – an eating pattern that cycles between periods of eating and not eating

Interferon – proteins that are part of the natural defences of the body

Intravenous infusions – the administration of fluids into a vein through a needle or catheter

Intuition – a form of knowledge that appears in consciousness without obvious deliberation

Iridology – the practice of studying the patterns and colours in the iris of the eye, to determine information about a person's health as a whole

Irritable Bowel Syndrome (IBS) – a disorder of the nerves and muscles of the large intestine causing pain and changed bowel habits

Jin Shin Yiutsu – a Japanese healing art that balances the energetic body, mind and spirit by using pressure points

Journaling – the practice of writing down thoughts and feelings for the purposes of self-analysis, self-discovery and self-reflection

Keratosis pilaris – a skin condition that causes small, hard bumps often called "chicken skin"

Kidneys – organs of filtration, filtering urine out of the blood

Kinesiologist – someone who specializes in the study of human movement, biomechanics

Kinesiology – a non-invasive holistic energy therapy, combining the ancient principles of Traditional Chinese Medicine (TCM) with modern muscle monitoring techniques

Leaky gut – gaps in the walls of the intestines that allow bacteria and other toxins to pass into the bloodstream

Lesion – an area of tissue that has been damaged through injury or disease

Ligament – fibrous connective tissue that connects bones to other bones

Lipoma – harmless, fatty lump that forms under the skin

Lobotomy - surgical severance of nerve fibres connecting the frontal lobes to the thalamus, to treat mental illness

Lupus – Systemic Lupus Erythematosus (SLE) – a chronic autoimmune disease which causes inflammation in connective tissues, affecting different body systems; joints, skin, kidneys, blood cells, brain, heart and lungs

Lyme disease – an infectious disease, spread by ticks, caused by a bacterium

Macrobiotic nutrition – a plant-based diet rooted in yin-yang theory from Asia

Mammogram – an X-ray image of women's breasts used to screen for breast cancer

Mantra – a mystical formula of invocation or incantation, of sounds, words or sentences

Massage – manipulation, by rubbing or kneading the body's soft tissues

Mastitis – an infection of breast tissue that most often occurs in women who breastfeed

McGill Pain Index – a scale that rates the level of pain

Meditation – an ancient mind/body technique that increases physical relaxation and enhances overall health and well-being

Menopause – the natural cessation of a woman's menstrual cycle; the end of fertility

Menstruation – the breaking down of the lining of the uterus which leaves the body through the vagina

Mental breakdown – a period of extreme mental or emotional stress

Meridian – channels through which qi (chi) flows, to nourish and energize the human body

Metaphysics – the seeking to understand the substance of reality: why things exist at all and what it means to exist in the first place

Microbiome – a collection of all microbes; bacteria, fungi, viruses and their genes, that naturally live on the inside and the outside surface the body

Migraine – a moderate to severe headache that often comes with nausea, vomiting, and sensitivity to light

Mindfulness – the practice of bringing conscious attention to experiences occurring in the present moment, without judgment

Miscarriage – a spontaneous abortion, loss of pregnancy

Mobile/mobility – the act of moving around

MRI – Magnetic Resonance Imaging is a technique using a magnetic field and computer-generated radio waves to create detailed images of the organs and tissues in the body

MTHFR gene mutation – inhibits the way the body processes folic acid and other important B vitamins, causing an increased risk for certain health issues

Multiple Myeloma – a cancer of plasma cells, a type of white blood cell that plays an important part in the immune system

Multiple Sclerosis (MS) – a disease of the central nervous system in which the insulating covers of nerve cells in the brain and spinal cord are damaged

Myalgic Encephalomyelitis (ME) – a debilitating, chronic condition that affects the nervous system, the immune system, and the body's production of energy

Myasthenia Gravis – a chronic autoimmune neuromuscular disease characterized by weakness of the skeletal muscles

Myers Cocktails – Intravenous therapy containing a solution of vitamins, minerals and nutrients

N-Acetylcysteine (NAC) – an antioxidant with numerous potential health benefits

Naturopath – person trained in the healing power of nature and the human body; treating the mind, body and spirit together

Neuro Linguistic Programming (NLP) – a way of changing someone's thoughts and behaviours to help achieve their desired outcomes

Neurologist – a medical doctor specialising in treating diseases of the nervous system

Neuropathy – damage or dysfunction of one or more nerves, causing tingling, numbness and pain

Nonverbal – little or no use of words or language

Nutritionist – a person who advises on matters of food and nutrition and their impacts on health

Obesity – an excessive amount of body fat

Occupational Therapist (OT) – a person who facilitates the participation in everyday living

Oesophagoscopy – a diagnostic procedure to check for abnormalities in the oesophagus

Oesophagus – a muscular tube from the throat to the stomach

Oestrogen/Estrogen – a hormone responsible for the development and regulation of the female reproductive system

Ophthalmologist – a physician specializing in the medical and surgical care of the eyes and vision

Orthostatic intolerance – an abnormal autonomic nervous system response when standing; symptoms of dizziness and fainting

Osteopenia – a condition in which bone mineral density is low

Osteoporosis – a disease that weakens bones

Palpitations – a feeling of a fast, heavy or fluttering heartbeat, can also be missed beats

Pancreas – an organ in the abdomen that helps in digestion of food and regulates blood sugar

Pancreatic cancer – cancer of the pancreas

Panic attack – sudden feelings of terror that come without warning

Paralysis – the loss of strength in and control over a muscle or group of muscles

Parasite – an organism that lives on or in a host and gets its food from or at the expense of its host

Parasite cleanse – diet, supplement, or other detox product that is intended to eliminate parasites from the body

Pathogens – organisms that cause disease

Periods – the regular discharge of blood and mucosal tissue from the inner lining of the uterus through the vagina, also known as menstruation

Pharmaceutical – a chemical substance used in healthcare

Physiokey – a bioadaptive impulse therapy device for the treatment of acute and chronic pain

Physiology – the study of how the human body works

Physiotherapy – treatment to restore mobility and normalcy in a patient's life

Phytonutrient – nutrients derived from plants

Phytotherapy – the use of molecules derived from plants for the treatment and prevention of disease

Plasma – the liquid portion of blood that is transports nutrients to the cells

Plasmapheresis – a procedure to remove some plasma from the blood

Poly-Cystic Ovarian Syndrome (PCOS) – a condition in which the ovaries produce an abnormal amount of male sex hormones

Post-Traumatic Stress Disorder (PTSD) – is a mental disorder which can develop after a person is exposed to a traumatic event

Postural Orthostatic Tachycardia Syndrome (POTS) – a disorder that can make someone feel faint or dizzy, caused by a problem with the autonomic nervous system (ANS)

Pranayama – breath control and the synchronising of the breath with movements

Prednisone – a medication used to suppress the immune system and reduce inflammation

Probiotics – living microorganisms that provide a health benefit when ingested

Progesterone – a female hormone important for the regulation of ovulation and menstruation

Prognosis – a prediction of the likely course and outcome of a disease

Prophylactic – a medication or a treatment to prevent a disease from occurring

Psychedelics/hallucinogens – a class of drug affecting all the senses, altering thinking, sense of time and emotions

Psychiatrist – a mental health doctor

Psychology – the scientific study of the mind and behaviour

Psychotherapy – using psychological techniques 'talk therapy' to encourage insight into problems

Radioactive Iodine therapy (RAI) – a treatment with radioactive iodide which is taken up in the thyroid gland where the radiation proceeds to destroy thyroid gland tissue

Rash – inflammation and/or discoloration that distorts the skin's normal appearance

Recall Healing – identifying and solving the emotional trauma behind a condition or behaviour

Rectal – relating to the rectum, the final straight portion of the large intestine before the anus

Reflexology – the application of appropriate pressure to specific points and areas on the feet, hands, or ears

Reflux/Heartburn – when stomach acid flows back up the food pipe, causing burning pain

Rehabilitation – treatment(s) designed to facilitate the process of recovery to as normal a condition as possible

Reiki – a Japanese form of alternative medicine called energy healing

Relaxation – a process that decreases the effects of stress on the mind and body

Restless leg syndrome – a nervous system disorder that causes an overpowering urge to move the legs

Reynard Disease – numbness, pain and discolouration in the hands or feet, caused by blood vessels overreacting to cold temperatures

Rheumatoid Arthritis – an autoimmune disease that causes chronic inflammation of joints

Rheumatologist – a doctor who specialises in diagnosing and treating inflammatory conditions affecting the joints, tendons, ligaments, bones, and muscles

Ringworm – a fungal infection of the skin, causing a circular rash

Sacral dimple – a dimple or indent, located at the end of the back, just above the crease of the buttocks, present at birth

Saliva – a clear liquid made by several glands in the mouth

Scabies – a contagious skin infection caused by a mite

Sciatica – pain caused by irritation, inflammation, pinching or compression of a nerve in the lower back

Sebaceous cyst – common noncancerous cysts of the skin

Seizures – changes in the brain's electrical activity causing noticeable symptoms or no symptoms

Self-Healing – the process of recovery, motivated by and directed by the person

Sensory – relating to the senses of hearing, touch, taste, smell and sight

Shaman – a person who acts as intermediary between the natural and supernatural worlds

Shiatsu – regulates the automatic nervous system activity and stimulates the circulatory system

Shingles – a viral infection that causes a painful rash, from the same virus that causes chickenpox

Shot – injection/vaccination

Sjögren's Syndrome – a systemic autoimmune disease affecting the entire body. Symptoms of extensive dryness, profound fatigue, chronic pain, major organ involvement, neuropathies and lymphomas

Smear/Pap test – a screening procedure for cervical cancer

Spider veins – small, thin veins that vary in colour, visible just under the surface of the skin

Spinal tap/Lumber puncture – a procedure to remove and test some of the cerebrospinal fluid around the spinal cord

Spirituality – an inward journey that involves a shift in awareness rather than some form of external activity

Spoonie – someone who suffers from a chronic illness

Stem Cells – primitive cells that have the potential to differentiate, or develop into, a variety of specific cell types

Stents – small mesh or plastic tubes that hold open passages in the body

Steroid – corticosteroids; to reduce inflammation and reduce the activity of the immune system – as creams, sprays, inhalers, tablets and injections

Strabismus – one eye is turned in a direction that is different from the other eye, also called crossed eyes

Streptococcal – a type of bacteria that can cause many different infections from minor illnesses to serious and deadly disease

Stress – the psychological perception of pressure and the body's response to it

Stroke – a lack of blood flow or a bleed, in the brain

Structured water – water with a structure that has been altered to form a hexagonal cluster

Subliminal – below the threshold of conscious perception

Sun spots – flat brown spots on the skin after sun exposure

Synergistic – different parts working together to produce an enhanced result

Tai-chi – a form of exercise based on martial arts involving slow movements and deep breathing

Taoism – a system of belief, attitudes and practices set towards the service and living to a person's nature

Temporomandibular joints syndrome – a disorder of the jaw muscles and nerves caused by injury or inflammation

Tendon – a tough band of fibrous connective tissue that connects muscle to bone

Thyroid – an endocrine gland in the neck which releases hormones that control metabolism

Tics – sudden, rapid, repetitive movements

Tinnitus – is the perception of noise or ringing in the ears when there is no noise

Tongue-tied – a condition present at birth that restricts the tongue's range of motion

Tonsillectomy – the surgical removal of the tonsils

Tonsils – small organs at the back of the throat, forming part of the lymphatic system

Touch of Matrix – a healing technique based on Quantum Physics for creating and transforming reality on the quantum level

Toxicity – the degree to which a chemical substance or a mixture of, can damage an organism

Toxicologist – someone who studies the presence and effects of toxins on humans

Toxin – a harmful/poisonous substance

Traditional Chinese Medicine (TCM) – a healing approach that originated in China using herbs, diet, acupuncture, cupping, and qigong to prevent or treat health problems, supporting physical, mental, emotional, and spiritual growth

Trans Ischaemic Attacks (TIA) – symptoms of a stroke but only lasting temporarily

Transcendental Meditation – a form of meditation that requires sitting for twenty minutes, twice a day and repeating a mantra, silently

Tremors – involuntary, rhythmic muscle contraction leading to shaking movements

Tumor/Tumour – an abnormal growth of cells that serves no purpose

Twelve step programme – a path to recovery from the abuse of drugs, alcohol or other behavioural disorders

Ulcer – a break or hole in a bodily membrane that impedes normal function of the affected organ

Ultrasound – high-frequency sound waves used to produce images of structures within the body

Urology – the field of medicine that focuses on diseases of the urinary tract

Vertigo – the sensation that either the body or the environment is moving

Visualization – the formation of mental visual image

Vitiligo – a disease that causes loss of skin colour, in patches

Vomiting – involuntary expulsion of the contents of the stomach, through the mouth (and nose)

Walk-in – a concept of a person whose original soul has departed their body and has been replaced with a new soul, either temporarily or permanently

Wheezing – a whistling sound that occurs during breathing

Yoga – an ancient practice that combines physical postures, breathing techniques and meditation or relaxation

Yogic – relating to the activity or philosophy of yoga

Zeolite – a natural, complex mineral used as a heavy metal detox supplement

Zumba – a fitness program consisting of dance and aerobic exercise routines performed to Latin American music